"Taylor and Colino have written the def
PMS. *Taking Back the Month* is a great re
cable research together with the real-life
who have found help. I do not know how anyone with PMS has man-
aged without this book. Neither will you."

—Rachel Naomi Remen, M.D.,
New York Times bestselling author

"Taking Back the Month is a breakthrough, non-drug approach to managing health and wellness in general and premenstrual symptoms in
particular. Dr. Taylor's insights are based on solid research . . . this
book will be a tremendous aid."

—Larry Dossey, M.D., author of
Healing Beyond the Body and *Healing Words*

"Bravo! Dr. Diana Taylor has rendered an immense service to all
women concerned with premenstrual symptoms, and the strategies she
recommends can be applied to every area of health and wellness. *Taking
Back the Month* will help anyone live a happier, more fulfilling life."

—Barbara Dossey, Ph.D.,
director, Holistic Nursing Association

"Taking Back the Month is a wonderful gift to women who experience
premenstrual symptoms. Dr. Taylor is giving back to women information that can change their everyday lives, their symptoms, well-being,
relationships, and their ability to function in the workplace. This is a
must-read for at least half of the population!"

—Nancy Fugate Woods, Ph.D., dean,
School of Nursing at University of Washington

"Taking Back the Month is unquestionably the most balanced and scientifically based of the available books about PMS. Dr. Taylor and Ms.
Colino have produced an engaging read that is full of important information, helpful advice, and therapeutic techniques that are easy to
understand and apply. Any woman who needs assistance in coping with
her premenstrual symptoms can surely find it here."

—Joan C. Chrisler, professor of psychology
at Connecticut College and president of the
Society for Menstrual Cycle Research

Taking Back the Month

A Personalized Solution for
Managing PMS and
Enhancing Your Health

Diana Taylor, R.N., Ph.D.,
and Stacey Colino

A Perigee Book

Every effort has been made to ensure that the information contained in this book is complete and accurate. However, neither the authors nor the publisher is engaged in rendering professional advice or services to the individual reader. The ideas, procedures, and suggestions contained in this book are not intended as a substitute for consulting with your physician. All matters regarding your health require medical supervision. Neither the authors nor the publisher shall be liable or responsible for any loss or damage allegedly arising from any information or suggestion in this book.

A Perigee Book
Published by The Berkley Publishing Group
A division of Penguin Putnam Inc.
375 Hudson Street
New York, New York 10014

Copyright © 2002 by Diana Taylor, R.N., Ph.D., and Stacey Colino
Text design by Tiffany Kukec
Cover design by Liz Sheehan
Cover art by Jose Ortega / SIS
Author photo of Diana Taylor copyright © Elena Dorfman, San Francisco
Author photo of Stacey Colino copyright © Goodman / Van Riper Photography

First edition: August 2002

Visit our website at www.penguinputnam.com

Library of Congress Cataloging-in-Publication Data

Taylor, Diana L.
    Taking back the month : a personalized solution for managing PMS and enhancing your health / by Diana Taylor and Stacey Colino.—1st ed.
        p.   cm.
    Includes bibliographical references and index.
    ISBN 0-399-52790-7
    1. Premenstrual syndrome.   2. Generative organs, Female—Diseases—Treatment.
I. Colino, Stacey.   II. Title.

RG165 .T385 2002
618.1'72—dc21
                                                                    2002025790

Printed in the United States of America

10 9 8 7 6 5 4 3 2 1

Contents

Acknowledgments

For both of us, this book has been a labor of love, and it would not have been possible without the assistance and influence of many people. First, we owe our thanks to the hundreds of women who have participated in the PMS Symptom Management Program at the University of California, San Francisco (UCSF) and the Oregon Health Sciences University (OHSU), women who shared their symptoms, their frustrations, and their lives. Ultimately, their experiences enabled us to show you how to create your own PMS solution. We also want to thank the informal participants—the many family members and friends—who've helped us to shape this program.

We are forever grateful to our agent, Michele Rubin, of Writers' House, who enthusiastically supported the concept behind this book from day one, and to our incredibly talented editor, Jennifer Repo, at Perigee, who wholeheartedly embraced this book and nurtured its development every step of the way.

At various stages of the writing process, several friends and colleagues read and commented on drafts—and helped us improve upon the original. In particular, we would like to thank Janis Jibrin, M.S., R.D. for her nutritional expertise; Dr. Nancy Woods who pioneered the research on PMS and perimenstrual symptoms; and Howard Robinson, Pharm.D., for his pharmacological review. We would also like to thank Claudia Schumann at the UCSF School of Nursing for her research assistance.

In addition, we each have our own mentors and personal supporters to thank.

From Diana:

First and foremost, I must recognize my coauthor, Stacey, who helped to make this project both fun and deeply gratifying. I would like to acknowledge the support from the National Institute of Nursing Research at the National Institutes of Health, which provided the funds to study the effectiveness of the PMS Symptom Management Program. And I would like to thank the Rockefeller Foundation's Bellagio Center, which provided support for the initial conceptualization of the project. I am grateful to Dr. Virginia Oleson who has inspired generations of researchers to think about women and their health beyond the confines of biomedicine. I am deeply indebted to my mentors at the University of Washington Center for Women's Health Research—Nancy Woods, Ellen Mitchell, and Marty Lentz—for their wisdom, vision, and professional guidance. A thank-you, also, to my friends and colleagues at the interdisciplinary Society for Menstrual Cycle Research—Ann Voda, Joan Chrisler, Kathleen MacPherson, Susan Cohen, Judy Berg, Jerilynn Prior, Alice Dan, Nancy Reame, Michelle Harrison, Jean Hamilton, and many other clinicians, researchers, and women's health advocates who have dedicated themselves to promoting research on the effects of the menstrual cycle on women's health across the lifespan. Special thanks go to Jay Welsh for his wise counsel and coaching, and to D'Anne Quinton and Jerry "the Sarge" Spolter for our weekly bicycle rides and their steadfast cheerleading. Additional recognition goes to Dean Kathleen Dracup, Dr. Betty Davies, and Brenda Roberts in the UCSF School of Nursing for their support and encouragement of this project.

I am deeply grateful to my husband, Jay Folberg, for his unwavering enthusiasm for this project as well as my work overall. His support sustains me and his gentle critique focuses my vision. And special thanks to my family who have been willing volunteers in crafting my early studies. To my children—Ross, Rachel, Lisa, and now our daughter-in-law, Lisa—who have provided me with a source of love and joy as well as research material over the years. Finally, a huge thank-you to my mother, sisters, sister-in-law, aunts, nieces, and girl-friends, who spent hours talking with me about their menstrual cycles, perimenstrual experiences, and health.

From Stacey:

I'm incredibly grateful to Diana for giving me the opportunity to write this book and for showing me how enormously rewarding it can be to work in a true collaborative spirit. My deep appreciation goes to the many family members and friends whose support and encouragement I came to rely upon during this project. In particular, I'd like to thank my mother, Willi Colino, my running partner and friend Nancy Petrisko, and Marie Park, Phyllis Jordan, Brian Wilson, and Nadine Schiavi for their kindness and generosity. Most of all, I'd like to thank my husband, Jon Fellner, and my son, Nate, for their ever-present love, patience, and inspiration, especially during the home stretch. The two of you make every month an absolute joy.

Introduction

Coming Unhinged

I *'m wrestling with temporary insanity.*
I've started calling myself Dr. Jekyll and Ms. Hyde.
I feel like I'm stuck in a black hole and I can't get out.
My life spins out of control for two weeks each month then I spend the next two weeks apologizing.
There are days when I'm better off staying away from people because I'm afraid of what I might say or do.

These are some of the ways in which women describe how they feel when they have premenstrual syndrome (PMS). Every month, almost like clockwork, women around the globe enter a period of time when they no longer feel like their usual selves. Suddenly, they're unable to stay on an even emotional keel, maintain their typical productivity at work, handle the various aspects of their lives comfortably, or relate to their families as they'd like to. Instead, they feel as though they're performing a high-wire act, trying to stay balanced and upright on a perilously thin foundation of support—from themselves and others.

Whether they are affected in body, mind, or both, countless women spend one-quarter to one-half of each month feeling drastically out of sorts. Over a woman's reproductive lifetime, this can add up to anywhere from nine to 18 years of feeling lousy as a result of premenstrual changes. Unfortunately, for many women, relief from these distressing symptoms has been extremely hard to come by.

For decades, the millions of women who suffer from PMS were told it was either all in their heads or something they'd need to learn to live with. Yes, it's true that PMS is in a woman's head—namely, in her pituitary gland and her hypothalamus—but it also resides in her adrenal glands and her ovaries, and it involves her autonomic and central nervous systems and probably her immune system, as well. Thanks to scientific research, it is now recognized that PMS is an actual mind/body condition with biological and behavioral roots, one that can produce a wide array of physical and emotional symptoms that can have a significant impact on a woman's life. While an estimated 50 to 75 percent of women experience some symptoms of PMS, approximately 5 to 10 percent of women suffer such profound depression, rages, and other extreme symptoms in the second half of the menstrual cycle that their ability to function basically screeches to a halt.

At the far end of this spectrum, the condition has been dubbed premenstrual dysphoric disorder (PMDD), a controversial label because it further medicalizes a natural phenomena in a negative way. PMDD is included in the latest *Diagnostic and Statistical Manual* (DSM-IV), the bible of psychiatric diagnoses, but many experts feel that there isn't sufficient research to support categorizing this condition as a psychiatric diagnosis. Plus, they feel that this amounts to pathologizing what is essentially a normal biological process and stigmatizing an entire gender because the mental disorder includes only women. On the positive side, a diagnosis of PMDD will improve the chances that women will get reimbursed by insurance companies for treatment.

Over the years, treatment for PMS has ranged from the dangerous (such as irradiation of the ovaries, shock therapy, or the use of leeches) to the ridiculous (such as hiding in one's room). Fortunately, women no longer have to suffer—or take refuge in the bedroom. With the benefit of new research, many new treatments have cropped up for PMS. And while there isn't a one-size-fits-all cure, a variety of promising remedies are available, and most women can find relief through a mix of approaches. Indeed, clinical research suggests that a customized combination of treatments may be more effective than any single one.

Nearly 20 years ago, I began working with women who have PMS.

Because I was a nurse practitioner, women told me about symptoms that seemed to recur around the time of menstruation, distressing symptoms that compromised their ability to function and the quality of their lives. Back then, few clinicians took these cyclical symptoms seriously; many of these women were simply referred for psychiatric treatment. Because so many women described similar symptom experiences, I began researching PMS and started a menstrual disorders program at the Oregon Health Sciences University in Portland. While looking for women to participate in a study, I placed an ad in a local newspaper and within a week received hundreds of phone calls in response. That's when I began to realize just how great a need there was for effective treatments for PMS.

In the past, research on PMS treatments has taken a scattershot approach at best. Researchers have tended to seize upon one possible solution—usually drugs—and investigated that exclusively or they've conducted studies that weren't well controlled. What was lacking was an integrated view of how to treat PMS—a big picture sense of treatments that might be effective and practical for women.

After obtaining a doctoral degree focused on women's health at the University of Washington in Seattle, I established a research program at the University of California, San Francisco (UCSF). I wanted to apply the same rigorous methods for studying drugs to the study of non-drug treatments for PMS. At the time, there were many untested treatments and home remedies. Women, however, wanted and needed scientific evidence about which remedies were merely folk cures, whether dietary changes work better than exercise, and whether there could be a one-size-fits-all treatment, as many other researchers have suggested. First, I collected information on all the non-drug treatments that had been recommended for PMS in the published medical literature. Then, I spoke to hundreds of women about these and other treatments they'd tried. What worked or didn't work for them? Which treatments were easier to sustain over the long term? What approaches made sense in the context of their lives?

These were among the questions I investigated while developing the UCSF PMS Symptom Management Program, a regimen of non-pharmacological strategies that involves self-monitoring, personal choice, self-regulation, and environmental modification. Over the years, more than 500 women have been studied and treated in my PMS

Symptom Management Programs, and it was a real education for me to guide them toward various interventions, keep track of their progress, and examine what worked for them. In the process, the PMS Symptom Management Program evolved as the stories and solutions of real women who suffered from PMS shed light on the steps that actually make a difference.

In collaboration with these women, I have created and tested a treatment protocol that reduces the severity of PMS and promotes general health and well-being for the vast majority of women who try it. On average, participants in the program at UCSF have experienced a 75 percent reduction in the intensity of their symptoms and a 30 to 54 percent reduction in feelings of depression and general distress in the premenstrual phase. And these were women with severe PMS, which suggests that women with mild to moderate PMS will obtain even greater results. In other instances, the program has helped women discover dual diagnoses—other health conditions that worsen premenstrually or that exist in conjunction with PMS and exacerbate it—that have made the premenstrual phase of their cycles that much harder to bear.

After hearing from hundreds of women about how helpful the UCSF PMS Symptom Management Program was, it seemed like a natural next step to turn this highly successful protocol into a program that women can use on their own, at home. This is usually where the story ends: Most research protocols, however successful they may be, don't venture beyond the walls of the ivory tower. This is where Stacey Colino, my coauthor, comes into the picture. An accomplished health writer and a strong advocate for consumer health, Stacey first helped me see how we might translate research protocols into user-friendly strategies that women could use on their own. Too often, researchers talk only to each other and become isolated and forget how to make our research findings come to life. My dream had always been to make my research relevant for real women but it took my collaboration with Stacey for this dream to become a reality. The symptom-management strategies you'll read about in this book are based on solid science, but without Stacey's background and her ability to take complex information and create step-by-step plans, the PMS Symptom Management Program would never have made it into something that every woman can use. Stacey's contribution to this project has been immense. As a woman with a family, a busy life, and a career, she has served as the conscience for women by providing regular reality checks to be sure various aspects of the program are pragmatic. She has also helped keep the voices of real women clear and present during the writing of this book. I am grateful for our partnership and I am certain that the PMS symptom management plan is all the better for it.

Rather than being a broad survey of PMS strategies from which women can randomly pick and choose, this program is a science-based protocol that has been proven to work for hundreds of women. This is not a cookie-cutter approach to curing PMS, as many other programs are. Too often women are told "change your diet," "reduce your stress," or "exercise"—but most treatment regimens don't include specific advice on how to achieve those goals. Nor are they individualized, depending on a woman's most bothersome symptoms and pressing needs. What women with PMS really want is a package of effective treatment strategies that suit their unique symptoms. This program offers that—and more.

In this book, you'll read about some of the treatments used in the UCSF PMS Symptom Management Program and learn how to try them on your own. We'll help you identify the symptoms that bother you the most and guide you in figuring out which lifestyle modifications or remedies are likely to work best to alleviate your discomfort. This way, you can discover the tools to help you experiment and see what works to relieve your premenstrual symptoms; in the process, you'll be enhancing your overall health physically, emotionally, behaviorally, and socially. You'll read the stories of women who participated in my PMS studies—though their names and identifying characteristics have been changed to protect their privacy—so that you can see how PMS affected their lives and what they did about it. As a woman doing research about women, I would never ask another woman to do something I wouldn't do. I have personally tested these strategies and so have my friends and family members (thank you, Lisa, Rachel, Linda, and Patty!).

At its core, this self-care program is really about identifying, controlling, and managing stress from the inside out and the outside in: Besides addressing specific symptoms of PMS, we'll help you pinpoint which aspects of your physical and social environments may be exacerbating your stress level and your symptoms. Then, we'll guide you toward strategies for managing difficult social situations and role conflicts. With our guidance, you'll be able to select the strategies that make the most sense for your life, which will help you custom-tailor a solution for your premenstrual misery and take back your life.

Diana Taylor, R.N., Ph.D.

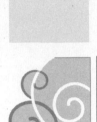

PART ONE

The Ups and Downs of PMS

1

The Puzzle of PMS

For years, it felt as though Samantha was looking for help in all the wrong places. In the early 1980s, she went to one doctor after another— internists, gynecologists, even psychiatrists—in a quest to obtain relief from the rapid mood swings, anxiety, sleep problems, food cravings, bloating, and cramps that ruled her life for nearly half of each month. She'd lash out angrily at her husband and often cry for no apparent reason. A senior attorney in a high-powered law firm, Samantha's symptoms were even beginning to take a toll on her performance at work: During the week before her period would arrive, she often had difficulty concentrating and would frequently become snippy with her colleagues.

"Most of the doctors I saw dismissed my symptoms as trivial," she recalls. "One physician I'd seen put me on thyroid medication, without doing any lab tests to see if I even had a thyroid problem. A psychologist I consulted suggested marital therapy. I was alternately angry and disappointed with the medical care I received."

Left to her own resources, Samantha, 31, began doing extensive research on PMS and became convinced that this was the source of her cyclical symptoms, which had suddenly appeared shortly after she suffered a miscarriage five years earlier. "Amazingly, only one of the many doctors I'd seen had ever heard of

PMS," she says. For more than two years, Samantha had tracked her symptoms—and found clear patterns that coincided with phases of her menstrual cycle—but none of the doctors would look at her records. "It was extremely frustrating," she says. "I had put a lot of things on hold until I could feel better. I'd even decided to put off having a baby because if I couldn't control my feelings and behavior then, how could I as a mother? I was afraid to be a mother with uncontrolled PMS. This was affecting my entire life and no one would take it seriously."

Contrary to once-popular belief, PMS isn't a figment of a woman's imagination, and it's not a form of mental illness, either. Women who experience PMS may feel as though they're suddenly losing their minds when, in fact, they may be psychologically healthy. They may feel quite ill for several days during their menstrual cycles when, in fact, they're actually in good physical health. Most bewildering of all, these women may feel quite normal for half the month, only to be overtaken by profound changes in their moods, physical equilibrium, or ability to conduct business as usual during the other half.

This is because PMS is a condition of complex origins—namely, neurological, hormonal, and behavioral interactions in the body—that can produce a wide array of physical and emotional symptoms. It typically occurs after ovulation through the first two to three days of a woman's period and can cause physical symptoms such as bloating, headache, weight gain, intestinal upset, sleep disturbances, breast tenderness, fatigue, and food cravings. In addition, PMS can trigger emotional or cognitive symptoms such as sudden mood swings, anxiety, anger, forgetfulness, depression, and a general feeling of being out of control. Behavioral changes—such as becoming argumentative or expressing anger more readily—are also common.

As it happens, more than 150 symptoms of PMS have been identified in the scientific and clinical literature. More often than not, women experience a combination of symptoms, usually a blend of emotional and behavioral changes such as irritability and crying jags or a combination of physical complaints such as pelvic cramps and backaches. Of course, many of these symptoms could occur because of other illnesses or conditions. What distinguishes them as part of PMS is their cyclical nature—the tendency to recur each month just before menstruation then to ease up after a woman's period begins. Here's a partial list of common symptoms that are associated with PMS:

Abdominal bloating	Impatience
Acne breakouts	Impulsiveness
Anger	Indigestion
Anxiety	Irritability
Awakening during the night	Joint pain or stiffness
Back- or neckache	Loneliness
Breast swelling and tenderness	Mood swings
Confusion	Muscle aches
Cramps (uterine or pelvic)	Nausea
Cravings	Nervousness
Crying spells	Night sweats
Depression	Numbness and tingling
Diarrhea	Out-of-control feelings
Difficulty concentrating	Panic
Difficulty falling asleep	Sex drive alterations
Dizziness	Shortness of breath
Eating more than usual	Skin disorder flare-ups
Fatigue or tiredness	Swelling of hands or feet
Forgetfulness	Tension
General aches and pains	Tremulousness/shakiness
Headaches	Vaginal dryness
Heart racing or pounding	Weight gain
Hot flashes	

To be considered premenstrual, these symptoms must occur regularly during the luteal phase—or second half of the menstrual cycle after ovulation occurs (following about day 14 in a 28-day cycle)—and they must be relieved by the onset of a woman's period or within a few days of the beginning of bleeding. In other words, a woman must have at least one week in which she is free of symptoms after her period ends in order for her symptoms to fall under the "premenstrual" umbrella. These time-sensitive and cyclical characteristics are what distinguish premenstrual symptoms from other gynecological or psychological conditions. The reason that PMS can have such far-reaching effects is that people have receptors for estrogen and progesterone—two of the hormones that are involved in PMS—throughout their entire bodies, as well as in the brain. That's why PMS can literally affect how a woman feels from head to toe.

Although the majority of women experience a few symptoms that are associated with the menstrual cycle's hormonal shifts—specifically, 95 percent of menstruating women will have one or more symptoms around the time of menstruation—up to 10 percent of menstruating women experience multiple symptoms to a severe degree. In addition, 25 to 40 percent of women in their reproductive years experience mild to moderate premenstrual symptoms, according to various studies. These numbers vary so widely because studies that have looked at the prevalence of PMS have used different methods or defined "symptoms" differently.

Generally, premenstrual symptoms refer to cyclical changes that a woman perceives as troublesome or problematic and that escalate before menstruation and then subside after a woman's period begins. Premenstrual symptoms of low to moderate intensity usually do not interfere with a woman's ability to function or perform her typical roles and, hence, they may not fall under the rubric of "premenstrual syndrome." They may constitute nothing more than premenstrual symptoms. Premenstrual syndrome (PMS), on the other hand, is a diagnostic term that's used to describe cyclical recurrences of distressing physical, emotional, and behavioral experiences that often affect a woman's relationships and personal health. A PMS symptom pattern can be discerned by the sudden absence of symptoms after a woman's period begins or by a low severity of symptoms after the onset of menstruation followed by an escalation of symptom frequency and severity during the premenstrual phase of her cycle. The hallmark of the syndrome is the repeated occurrence of physical, emotional, and behavioral symptoms that are severe enough to alter a woman's ability to function socially or occupationally during the premenstrual phase of her cycle. But it's the severity, the number, and the duration of symptoms that affect the intensity of the premenstrual stew.

Depending on its severity, the disorder can disrupt nearly every aspect of a woman's life—her work and home life, her relationships with family members and friends, the way she eats and sleeps, and so on—profoundly or mildly. Several studies have found that women report greater difficulties concentrating during the premenstrual and/or menstrual phases, although these variations have not been measured objectively. Whether it's due to a woman's perception of her abilities or to actual changes in her cognitive function, severe cases of PMS have been found to reduce a woman's efficiency at work and increase absenteeism. In my own studies of women with severe PMS, 50 percent of the women said their work productivity was affected by their symptoms for anywhere from two to 20 days during the previous three months. On average, the women felt their ability to concentrate, organize their work, or be efficient was hindered approximately three days per month, regardless of the nature of their work. Meanwhile, about a third of the women with severe PMS reported one to ten days of work were missed because of their symptoms in the previous three months.

The Causal Conundrum

While it is widely accepted that PMS is related to hormonal changes during the menstrual cycle, the exact cause still remains a mystery. Over the years, biological theories have pointed to an excess of estrogen, a deficiency of progesterone, an imbalance between estrogen and progesterone, an increase in aldosterone (a hormone that's secreted by the adrenal gland and acts on the kidney to regulate salt and water balance), low blood sugar, and an excess of the hormone prolactin (which stimulates progesterone production by the ovary as well as milk production after pregnancy) as possible causal factors. Others have suggested that vitamin or mineral deficiencies—in particular, low levels of vitamin B-6 and more recently a calcium deficiency—may contribute to PMS.

Meanwhile, other researchers have examined the association between PMS and personality attributes, coping style, and acceptance or rejection of a woman's role in society. Still other researchers suspect that premenstrual mood swings may stem from changes in the brain's chemistry—namely, from a drop in the feel-good brain chemical serotonin—that occur in response to these monthly hormonal fluctuations. Some investigators have even suggested that the mood aspects of PMS constitute a form of atypical depression.

Another body of research suggests that stress may be a contributing or exacerbating factor. It could be that women who feel perpetually stressed-out perceive their health more negatively—or that this state of chronic stress may spark an increase in premenstrual symptoms. Granted, experiencing premenstrual symptoms that are severe enough to compromise a woman's ability to function is a source of stress in itself, which could create a vicious cycle of stress and symptoms. In my own research, I have found that women with severe PMS experience a moderate to high degree of stress, primarily work- and home-related stress, during the premenstrual phase. These effects can be far-reaching. After all, stress isn't only a matter of perception: In the midst of stress, the body's fight-or-flight response is sparked, which leads to increased secretion of various hormones including cortisol, epinephrine, and aldosterone. In addition, stress can disrupt the body's balance of estrogen and progesterone—all of which can amplify a woman's premenstrual symptoms and her reaction to stress.

As scientists continue to untangle and investigate the intricate array of factors that may play a role in PMS, the actual experience of PMS remains unchanged for women as a whole. And the truth is, there isn't likely to be one general theory that explains the flare-up of premenstrual symptoms for all women. Currently, the prevailing view is that women with PMS are simply more sensitive to what are essentially normal hormonal shifts and, as a result, they wind up with symptoms that don't affect other menstruating women. In fact, some of these physiological changes may make more of a difference for some women who experience PMS than others: It may be that one woman is particularly sensitive to premenstrually induced low blood sugar, whereas another might be hypersensitive to changes in serotonin levels. Perhaps changes in the levels of gonadal steroids that are released by the pituitary gland trigger a change in a woman's mood—or otherwise predispose her to mood instability—in those who are sensitive to these particular hormones. Or it could be that a woman's response to stress is a key factor, which has an impact on her blood sugar levels and so on.

It's a synergistic response between biology and behavior, in which some of these changes may be more pronounced in a woman with PMS or in which she has a heightened response to these normal physiological changes. Moreover, it may be that women with PMS have trouble coping with these physiological shifts as well as with other stressful aspects of their lives, which can exacerbate the intensity of premenstrual symptoms. It's a delicate pas de deux between mind and body—and how a woman performs under these conditions depends largely on her personal vulnerability to these changes.

The Phases of Your Cycle

Since PMS occurs in the context of menstruation, it helps to understand the anatomy of the menstrual cycle itself. The menstrual cycle is not simply switched on at menarche (the onset of menstruation, usually around age 12 or 13) and switched off at menopause (the cessation of menstruation, usually between the ages of 45 and 55). It is a many-faceted biological process that has a starting phase (menarche), a phase of optimal operation (during the childbearing years), and a phase of decline (known as the perimenopause), until it ceases completely (menopause).

In the intervening years, the menstrual cycle, a biological phenomenon with an ebb and flow of physical and psychological effects, is an important part of being female. The menstrual cycle is not the same as a menstrual period. A menstrual period consists of the days that a woman bleeds as the uterus sheds its lining. The menstrual cycle, by contrast, is the span of time from the start of one menstrual period to the start of

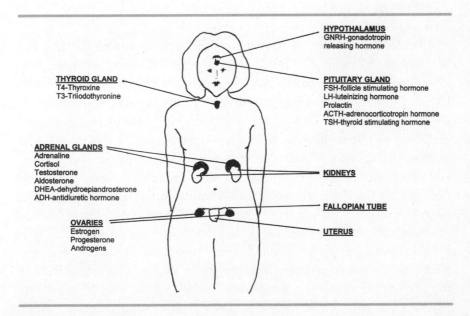

FIGURE 1.1

Hormone Secreting Glands and Major Sources of Hormones in a Woman's Body

the next. During the menstrual cycle, low levels of one hormone stimulate rising levels of another, creating a continuous pattern of rising and falling hormones that repeats itself on a monthly basis. The cycle is initiated and maintained by the rhythmic activity of the ovaries, which give rise to changing levels of pituitary and ovarian hormones.

Most women who menstruate normally will have a somewhat predictable cycle, with four phases that add up to about 28 days each month (sometimes referred to as the "lunar month"), although the menstrual cycle can vary from 25 to 35 days. The four primary phases of the menstrual cycle typically occur as follows, using a 28-day cycle as an example:

Menstrual phase=Days 1–5

Follicular phase=Days 6–12 (also referred to as the postmenstrual phase)

Ovulatory phase=Days 13–15

Luteal phase=Days 16–28 (also referred to as the premenstrual phase)

Technically, day one of your menstrual cycle occurs on the first day of menstrual bleeding. After a woman's period ends, the hormones estrogen and progesterone, which are made by the ovaries, cause changes in the lining of the uterus; this is called the follicular phase of the menstrual cycle. This is the most variable phase of the menstrual cycle and can be as short as five to seven days (in a 21-day cycle) or as long as 20 days (in a 35-day cycle). In the meantime, a number of ovarian follicles (or eggs) start to mature, one of which is released at ovulation (a.k.a., the ovulatory phase), on about day 14 (in a 28-day cycle). After ovulation, which is also known as the luteal phase, the reciprocal relationship between ovarian and pituitary hormones provides the basis for the formation of the corpus luteum (a cellular structure that produces high levels of estrogen and progesterone) and the preparation of the uterus (the womb) for pregnancy. If the egg (or follicle) is not fertilized by a sperm, the corpus luteum begins to degenerate, which causes levels of estrogen and progesterone to decrease.

Ultimately, this withdrawal of hormonal support prompts the uterus to shed its lining (or endometrium). The time period from ovulation to the onset of your period is called the luteal phase of the menstrual cycle, which typically lasts 14 days in a normal menstrual cycle. When the uterus sheds its lining, menstrual bleeding (a.k.a., your period) occurs, which designates the start of a new cycle. While an ovulatory menstrual cycle can be quite variable, we will use the 28-day cycle that's often described for the sake of simplicity. (If your cycle is longer or shorter, the phases of your cycle will likely correspond accordingly.)

Whether the severity of PMS symptoms is related to longer menstrual cycles—31 to 40 days, in particular—has been much debated. In fact, several studies have failed to show a relationship between the length of the menstrual cycle and the level of distress caused by symptoms. Other variations in the length of menstrual cycles produce more predictable effects on premenstrual symptoms. Women with short, irregular ovulatory cycles, for example, have the highest incidence of both premenstrual and menstrual symptoms. Unfortunately, this means that since the premenstrual phase remains constant—lasting 14

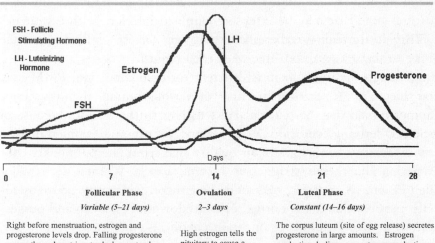

FSH - Follicle Stimulating Hormone

LH - Luteinizing Hormone

Estrogen

LH

Progesterone

FSH

Days

0   7   14   21   28

Follicular Phase   **Ovulation**   **Luteal Phase**

Variable (5–21 days)   *2–3 days*   *Constant (14–16 days)*

Right before menstruation, estrogen and progesterone levels drop. Falling progesterone causes the endometrium to shed; menstrual bleeding occurs. The pituitary secretes FSH to stimulate follicles (eggs) inside the ovary to develop and secrete more estrogen. The follicular phase is variable—14 days in a 28-day cycle; 21 days in a 35-day cycle but only 7 days in a 21-day cycle.

High estrogen tells the pituitary to cause a surge in LH, which triggers ovulation; an egg erupts from a follicle into a fallopian tube.

The corpus luteum (site of egg release) secretes progesterone in large amounts. Estrogen production declines; progesterone production rises further. The corpus luteum gradually deteriorates if the egg is not fertilized. Cramping and uterine contractions occur as both estrogen and progesterone levels decline; menstruation occurs. The luteal phase is relatively constant, lasting approximately two weeks.

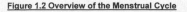

Figure 1.2 Overview of the Menstrual Cycle

to 16 days from ovulation to the onset of menses—and the menstrual phase lasts about three to five days, a woman with a 20 to 25 day menstrual cycle might have only one to five symptom-free days each month. Meanwhile, women whose menstrual cycles last longer than 40 days usually report few premenstrual symptoms. This may be because there's a good chance these women have anovulatory cycles—meaning, they aren't ovulating—which produces fewer premenstrual symptoms.

Adding Insult to Misery

Besides sparking symptoms directly, premenstrual changes also can aggravate underlying health conditions such as asthma and allergies, depression, herpes, sinusitis, and irritable bowel syndrome (IBS), among others, or make it more difficult to manage these conditions. This is called *premenstrual magnification* (PMM), and it is defined as an underlying problem that worsens during the premenstrual phase (meaning 7 to 14 days before the onset of menstruation). This is a variant of the PMS pattern in which women experience moderately severe symptoms after their periods start and more severe symptoms beforehand. In other words, PMM is a cyclical flare-up of an underlying condition—one that may be intense enough to interfere with a woman's ability to function—rather than the usual pattern of PMS since she may not have a symptom-free week each month.

Though the mechanism is different for each condition, PMM may be due to the trickle-down effect of various hormonal fluctuations. Some women may be particularly sensitive to these shifts because of their underlying condition. With asthma, for example, women may be more sensitive to changes in air quality that stimulate pulmonary constriction and thereby trigger an asthma attack. Women with major depression, by contrast, may find their mood worsening premenstrually, possibly due to the normal ups and downs of estrogen and progesterone and their influence on brain chemicals such as serotonin. Yet, many women don't make the connection between flare-ups of these conditions and the hormonal fluctuations that are associated with PMS. Or, if they haven't been diagnosed with the underlying problem, they may think their symptoms simply reflect PMS when they actually suggest that something else is going on, as well.

Most women who monitor their experiences on a daily basis over the course of more than one menstrual cycle notice changes in their bodies and moods that seem to vary with the course of the menstrual cycle. These can range from what could be considered normal menstrual experiences to illness-like symptoms, from mild premenstrual changes to premenstrual syndrome. Many women who experience changes such as swelling of their breasts or abdomen, menstrual cramps, or bursts of energy do not consider themselves sick or ill. Instead, they view such changes as a "natural" part of being a woman—and they deal with them matter-of-factly and don't seek medical care.

Premenstrual changes aren't a guaranteed negative state for all women but it may surprise you to learn that some women describe *positive* experiences that are associated with shifts in the menstrual cycle: These might include an increased energy level or heightened creativity or a surge of self-confidence or sexual desire at various phases of their cycles. In a study of women without PMS, researchers at Connecticut College found that when the concept of "menstrual joy" was introduced in a questionnaire before administration of a menstrual distress questionnaire and a menstrual attitude questionnaire, women reported more positive attitudes toward menstruation and more positive ratings of cyclical changes. It wasn't that their periods had become altogether blissful experiences; rather, these women had simply begun to notice the positive effects their cycles had on their lives. In the premenstrual phase, for instance, many of the women experienced increased sexual desire, feelings of affection, and self-confidence. After the study, 30 percent of the participants said the menstrual joy questionnaire caused them to look at menstruation in a different light.

The Many Faces of PMS

At some point during their lifetimes, the majority of all women will experience menstrual-related symptoms that will require professional treatment or self-management. While the most common reported premenstrual symptoms may be complaints of physical discomfort (bloating, skin changes, cramping, and the like), the mood changes or negative-affect symptoms—anxiety, tension, depression, etc.—are often the most distressing to women. In a healthy, community-based sample of 193 women from a southeastern U.S. city, the most prevalent premenstrual symptoms were cramps, mood swings, fatigue, swelling, irritability, tension, skin disorders, headache, depression, backache, painful or tender breasts, weight gain, anxiety, and crying. In another study of 345 women from diverse ethnic backgrounds on the West Coast, the symptoms the women most frequently rated as moderate or extreme during the premenstrual phase of their cycles were fatigue, sensation of weight gain, awakening during the night, depression, painful or tender breasts, and bloating.

Yet, the emotional changes are often the most distressing because they can make a woman feel frazzled and out of control—as if she's becoming someone she doesn't want to be. After all, successful women should be perfectly calm, cool, and composed all the time, right? PMS often throws a wrench in that possibility.

"What bothers me the most is the rage that builds inside me," confesses Ellen, 32, a physical therapist and mother of a toddler. "For a few days before my period, I can't seem to control my feelings or what I say or do. I yell and scream at my son and my husband over the smallest thing. My son spills his milk; my husband doesn't come home the exact minute he tells me he'll be there—and I go berserk. It scares me to feel this way. Sometimes, when my period comes, I cry from relief, just knowing that these intense feelings are over for a while."

Because so many symptoms have been attributed to shifts in the menstrual cycle, several researchers have focused on identifying symptom clusters. After all, it is not unusual for a woman with PMS to experience as many as ten symptoms in a particular month. This delineation of symptoms into clusters has helped clinicians understand women's full experience of premenstrual symptoms, rather than focusing on symptoms in a piecemeal fashion. It has also helped us direct women toward appropriate treatments for managing their symptoms.

In general, most premenstrual symptoms can be clustered into one of four groups:

Pain/discomfort symptoms, which include abdominal/pelvic pain, headaches, joint aches and pains, back and neckache, and the like.

Somatic/cognitive symptoms, which include physical symptoms such as constipation, nausea, gas, acne, itching, weight gain, fatigue, forgetfulness, and poor judgment.

Behavioral/functional changes, including increased appetite, food cravings, acting impulsively, poor coordination, decreased efficiency, and lowered work performance.

Mood-related symptoms, which are the most common cluster, account for 60 percent of the complaints in my research. These can actually be subdivided into two clusters: "Turmoil," which includes feelings of anxiety, anger, nervousness, restlessness, and oversensitivity; and "the blues," which includes feeling sad, lonely or depressed, crying easily, and a low self-image.

Granted, a woman may not have every symptom in a particular cluster and her symptoms may fluctuate somewhat from one month to the next. But she may find that the majority of her complaints—or perhaps her most irritating symptoms—tend to fall in a particular cluster and that each of these symptoms ebbs and flows across the menstrual cycle. Recognizing this can help her choose her treatments accordingly.

PREMENSTRUAL DYSPHORIC DISORDER

While many people believe that PMS and PMDD (premenstrual dysphoric disorder) are synonymous, this is simply not the case. PMDD is a diagnostic label that applies to a smaller number of menstruating women—no more than 8 percent—and includes more severe premenstrual symptoms. It was initially labeled "late luteal phase dysphoric disorder" in 1987 but was changed in 1994. While PMS may be like having a few days of thunderstorms each month, PMDD is more like a hurricane that keeps circling around and continuously tearing apart the emotional foundation of your life for up to two weeks. There's no question that some women experience a more severe form of PMS. It's the marketing of a disorder that troubles many feminists and medical scholars: By including PMDD as a diagnosis in the DSM-IV and classifying it among major mood disorders, the concern is that this is legitimizing PMDD or severe PMS as a psychiatric disorder.

The makers of Sarafem, a new packaging of Prozac specifically for PMDD (by Eli Lilly), then use this relatively new classification to sell more of the drug, even though there's no magic bullet for any form of PMS. It's an example of what psychologist Paula Caplan, Ph.D., of

Brown University, has dubbed "the drug in search of a disease" phenomenon that is overtaking the pharmaceutical industry. After all, PMS is a complex condition that can take many shapes in different women. And the reality is, no single treatment will address all of these facets.

While Sarafem may ease some of the insomnia and mood symptoms that are associated with PMS, it won't have any effect on physical symptoms such as pain, bloating, and so on. Plus, many of the selective serotonin reuptake inhibitors (SSRIs), including Prozac, can quash a woman's libido, which could create another problem if PMS is already straining her romantic relationship. Moreover, research has found that 40 percent of women with PMS don't respond to Prozac and other SSRIs. Which means that a substantial proportion of women with this condition are left out in the cold, even though Sarafem has been billed as a cure-all for PMS. The truth is, as much as women (and the pharmaceutical industry) might wish it were so, there isn't a pill that's a panacea for PMS.

CULTURAL VARIATIONS ON A THEME

Interestingly, certain symptoms appear to be more common among different cultures. In a cross-cultural study from the early 1970s, researchers assessed the incidence of premenstrual syndrome among six cultural groups—American, Japanese, Nigerian, Apache, Turkish, and Greek. What they found is that, overall, Turkish women reported the highest incidence of all premenstrual physical and mood symptoms, whereas Japanese women reported the lowest incidence of premenstrual symptoms. When it comes to mood symptoms—including irritability, depression, tension, and being easily upset—Turkish and American women were most similar. About half of Apache women reported experiencing depression and irritability, and approximately 63 percent reported feeling tension and being easily upset. Greek women reported the highest incidence of premenstrual depression—78 percent of the women reported it—whereas only about 40 percent of Japanese women report premenstrual depression.

What accounts for all these cultural differences in the experience of premenstrual symptoms? No one knows for sure. But what is known is that PMS is not a generic experience: Each woman experiences her own version of the phenomenon, and her experience may be influenced by a variety of factors, including cultural attitudes, her socioeconomic and/or marital status, how many children she has, and her education level. While the experience of menstrual cyclicity certainly seems to have cultural variations, premenstrual syndrome (PMS) itself is a medically constructed phenomenon. First defined by Dr. Robert T. Frank, of the U.S., as premenstrual tension in 1931 and later by Dr. Katharina Dalton, a British physician, as premenstrual syndrome in 1953, this term has no equivalent in many other cultures.

Moreover, cultural and social beliefs influence the cognitive and emotional processing of these changes and, hence, the experience. If a woman grows up in Turkey, for example, and nobody there talks about depression before menstruation but people do talk about bloating and tension, that's what she may be likely to focus on. It may not be that Turkish women don't experience the pre-period blues; it simply may be that they're not attuned to these psychological changes. In other words, attitudes toward menstruation may be culturally or socially transmitted, to some degree, from the time girls first begin to menstruate.

THE EFFECTS OF NOT-SO-GREAT EXPECTATIONS

For the most part, people in the U.S. tend to harbor negative associations with menstruation, views that are often fueled by the media. When analyzing the content of magazine articles about PMS that were published between 1980 and 1987, researchers at Connecticut College found that most articles were negative in their tone and supported the stereotype of the woman who experiences PMS as a maladjusted woman. Whether this influence is subtle or overt, it can have a mighty influence on women's experience of premenstrual changes. Negative menstrual attitudes promoted by society form a type of cultural straitjacket, constricting a woman's emotional and intellectual growth—and her experience of her body.

Beliefs and expectations about menstruation and premenstrual symptoms can be transmitted in various ways—through the media, by health professionals, and through family members and peers. Young girls, for instance, learn about premenstrual symptoms from observing their mothers, sisters, and friends, and these observations can, in turn, affect their own feelings and behavior as they begin to menstruate. Indeed, research has found that mothers' experiences with premenstrual symptoms appear to be linked to daughters' subsequent symptom experiences. Researchers at the University of Washington in Seattle have found that women with PMS and premenstrual magnification (PMM) symptom patterns were more likely to have had a mother with more premenstrual symptoms than women who experienced few symptoms in conjunction with the menstrual cycle.

If anyone can attest to the relationship between family ties and PMS, it's Melanie, 48, and her 20-year-old daughter Carolyn. From the age of 20, Melanie had experienced bloating, shakiness, nervousness, headaches, insomnia, overeating, and hot flashes nearly every month for the ten days before the arrival of her period—a pattern that continued for more than 25 years. Unfortunately, Carolyn followed in her mother's footsteps and also struggled with bloating, hot flashes, insomnia, and irritability for about ten days each month. This didn't come as a complete surprise to Carolyn, especially since she'd grown up hearing her mother gripe about her period. "I was always aware of my mother's PMS, and my brother and I used to stay away from her when she got that way," Carolyn admits. "Now I know how she feels—like an ogre or guilty for saying things she didn't mean."

Whether this mother-daughter link is due to socially transmitted attitudes or to genetic similarities between mothers and daughters remains unclear. What is apparent is that the expectation-experience link can create a perpetuating cycle: While women may come to expect premenstrual symptoms for a variety of reasons, their actual experience of symptoms can also come to influence their expectations. In other words, women who have premenstrual symptoms may come to anticipate their arrival each month and, hence, may perceive events around the time of menstruation as more stressful. And this heightened perception of stress may wind up exacerbating their symptoms and so on.

In recent years, the prevailing American medical model of PMS, which focuses on the negative symptoms women "suffer," has been exported to other countries and cultures. It appears that women in other cultures who have been exposed to the notion of "PMS as a disease" or to health-related information that promotes a physical cause for unavoidable mood and cognitive symptoms that are associated with the menstrual cycle may be more likely to report negative symptoms. Certainly, women with more education and more access to the media, regardless of their ethnicity or culture, are more heavily exposed to this negative view of PMS. As unfortunate as this is, the fact that beliefs and expectations about premenstrual changes are learned offers a note of optimism as well: If women are provided with a more favorable view of these cyclical shifts, perhaps they will begin to perceive or experience them in a more positive light. This can actually be achieved with the use of cognitive strategies that are designed to alter the way a woman views such experiences. (You'll read more about this in Chapter Seven, "Giving Your Mindset a Makeover.")

GETTING TO THE BOTTOM OF THE MATTER

Even though there aren't any physical, hormonal, or psychological tests to gauge if a woman has PMS, most women believe they know if they've experienced the syndrome. This is one of those situations in life where you might think you would know it if you saw it or felt it. But it's so critical to chart your own symptoms because it is possible to be fooled by your own body: If, for example, you have alternating bouts of diarrhea and constipation premenstrually you might think it's PMS when these symptoms could be signs of irritable bowel syndrome. Or, you might discover, in the course of charting your symptoms, that your flare-ups don't actually correspond to a particular point in your menstrual cycle. As you've already seen, the essential element for PMS is that the symptoms that exist in the premenstrual phase of your cycle ease up considerably or disappear altogether with the onset of your period. Another essential element is that these symptoms recur with some regularity, even if they don't reappear every single month.

In a sense, you're the most qualified expert to detect clues that you may have PMS. By charting your symptoms in exquisite detail over a few months, you'll become keenly aware of what a normal menstrual cycle is for you and which symptoms tend to occur in a cyclical fashion. (You'll learn how to track these factors in Chapter Three, "Getting in Touch with Your Symptoms.") Once you've recorded your pattern of daily symptoms along with their severity for two or three cycles, you'll be in a better position to rule out other chronic illnesses that might vary with the menstrual cycle. You'll also be able to take an unvarnished look at whether you have full-blown PMS or simply a few irritating premenstrual symptoms. This will help you figure out what steps to take so that you'll feel better all month long.

2

The Ages and Stages of PMS

When her period first arrived in its crimson glory, Charlotte was 12 and considered herself lucky because she suffered only menstrual cramps, not the debilitating PMS that her mother had been complaining about for years. Within two years, however, Charlotte began experiencing headaches, bloating, sleep disturbances, mood swings, food cravings, and acne flare-ups about ten days before the start of her period. The symptoms would typically disappear on the first day of bleeding, only to reappear again and again often in a more severe incarnation. "My symptoms have definitely gotten worse as I've gotten older," says Charlotte, now 18, a college student. "When I'm premenstrual, I'm cranky, restless, and impatient with everything and everybody, and I can't get as much work done as I'd like to. I dread these times, especially if I'm trying to get ready for a test or a paper."

Vicki's introduction to PMS was quite different. During her early menstrual years, she didn't experience any premenstrual symptoms and her period didn't particularly bother her, either. All that changed when she reached her mid-thirties, when suddenly depression, lethargy, irritability, mental dullness, and cramping began to strike each month during the period before her period. Over the years, Vicki's emotional symptoms, in particular, worsened. It got to the point where she'd spend ten to 15 days feeling just plain lousy. "I loathe this time of the month," admits Vicki, 45, an office manager. "I feel depressed and withdraw from the world. My work productivity suffers. My social life is affected. And my boyfriend accuses me of not trying hard enough to control the symptoms." Once she became perimenopausal, her menstrual cycles shortened to about 25 days, which meant that she had only five to seven symptom-free days each month.

Sadly, these women's experiences are not a fluke, because PMS is not always a predictable or linear condition. It can come and go from one month to the next. It can occur for the first time or worsen during certain phases of a woman's life. And it can flare up during periods of physical or psychological stress. And when the source of that stress eases up, PMS may or may not retreat.

Even in relatively calm times, some premenstrual phases are likely to be worse than others, and a woman's symptoms may be quite different from her friends' or family members'—and this is quite normal. After all, everyone responds to environmental and hormonal stimuli quite differently, both physically and emotionally. Individual symptoms may vary from month to month because certain body systems may be more sensitive to particular stimuli at some times than others. Subtle hormonal variations from one month to the next, for example, can trigger different symptoms or a different intensity of the same symptoms in a particular woman. And when a woman is enduring a prolonged bout of stress—for example, during final exams in college—or a phase of major physical and psychological adjustment, as with perimenopause, premenstrual symptoms can become magnified and often that much harder to endure.

Who's Vulnerable—and Why

The reality is, young girls who haven't begun to menstruate don't have PMS, and neither do women who've gone through menopause. Premenstrual symptoms are naturally and inextricably connected to a woman's menstrual cycle so they occur only while a woman is considered to be of reproductive age—meaning, as long as she has a period and is capable of becoming pregnant. But it's not the hormonal highs or lows that ignite PMS. Research suggests that it's the change in hormone levels, rather than the absolute levels of hormones, that triggers symptoms in women who are susceptible to PMS.

Of course, a rapid change in ovarian hormone levels is not unique to the premenstrual phase of the menstrual cycle. Even more dramatic changes occur in the postpartum period, which is why many women experience a temporary period of sadness or "the baby blues" within the first ten days of giving birth. In this instance, too, not every woman will experience these symptoms: Only those who are vulnerable to these hormonal fluctuations do. Similar mood changes can occur during adolescence, the first trimester of pregnancy, and the perimenopause. The common denominator in all of these time periods is an increased variability in hormonal levels and, perhaps, an increased sensitivity to these shifts, among some women.

Because all menstruating women experience these cyclical shifts in hormones, and because not all women experience premenstrual symptoms, there must be some explanation for why some women will have symptoms and others under the same biological circumstances will not. One theory is that certain women may be personally vulnerable—physically, emotionally, behaviorally, and socially—to these changes at some times in their lives and perhaps not others. Rather than being a static, predetermined state, this vulnerability is a fluid, dynamic process in which personal experiences come into play. In the context of premenstrual symptoms, vulnerability has been defined as "a mutually amplifying interaction" between hereditary factors, life events and a woman's perception of them, and underlying levels of functioning and symptoms at the time of a particular change.

Even before birth, for example, the genetic tendency toward PMS may be established by hormonal influences that may not become apparent until later stages of life. Early experiences can also shape a woman's vulnerability if, as a teenager, she develops a particular pattern of response (such as dread) to her period. If a woman has trouble coping with premenstrual symptoms when they do appear, this can increase her vulnerability even more in the future. In addition, the normal aging process physically contributes to a woman's increased vulnerability as she gets older, simply because of the wear and tear on her body and the natural hormonal shifts that occur with the passing years. Over time, impairment of the body's natural state of balance (or homeostasis) which occurs with high levels of stress or repeated cycles of premenstrual symptoms can increase a woman's vulnerability to PMS by acting as a sensitizing "kindling" process: With repeated stress or physiologic changes, it may take less and less to trigger a woman's premenstrual symptoms.

Normally, during the premenstrual period, levels of several hormones such as estrogen and progesterone, along with other substances in the body such as neurotransmitters like dopamine and norepinephrine fluctuate widely but in a way that's balanced and in harmony. If the pace and level of change between these key hormones are relatively similar, then few or no premenstrual changes will occur. On the other hand, if these hormones and other substances change rapidly but at different paces and levels, homeostasis between hormones, modulators, neurotransmitters, and bodily processes will be temporarily impaired. In this case, a woman's vulnerability to external stimuli may be increased but still she may perceive her premenstrual symptoms as minimally distressing. This often happens to adolescents who have begun to menstruate but haven't developed negative expectations about their periods or the premenstrual phase of their cycles. It can also happen to women as they enter perimenopause if they don't have a history of PMS.

It's when a variety of factors conspire that a woman becomes truly vulnerable to PMS: If the homeostasis is disrupted and a woman's hormones change rapidly at different paces and levels and she's under stress and she typically has negative associations with the phase before her period, then she's likely—or "highly vulnerable"—to experience bothersome premenstrual symptoms. In addition, women who have certain chronic health conditions—such as asthma, epilepsy, or panic disorders—are at increased risk for flare-ups of these conditions premenstrually because they're entering a biologically vulnerable time. All of these cyclical amplifications may contribute to an increased incidence and severity of premenstrual changes with advancing age. (A note of good news: This mechanism doesn't have to be self-perpetuating; a variety of therapies can restore this homeostatic balance, as you'll see in the chapters that follow.)

Surprisingly enough, some women respond to these premenstrual changes in a certain way for a few years then all of a sudden they might start having different symptoms—and it isn't always known why. It's not likely to be a simple process because PMS involves a complex interaction between the woman and her environment with all its varying facets. Usually women will have a similar constellation of symptoms for a while. One woman might experience anxiety, irritability, water retention, and sleep problems, for example; another might have tension, headaches, food cravings, and fatigue. Depending on which ovary they ovulate from, they might have a different balance of hormones in a particular month, which can affect the severity of their symptoms. Many women will ovulate from the same ovary each month (we usually have one dominant ovary, and sometimes the other one acts as a spare tire), but some women will go back and forth between the ovaries. When that happens, a woman's premenstrual symptoms are likely to vary in severity from one month to another. Even among those who have true PMS, the symptoms may be mild or severe or vary between the two extremes from month to month or from one stage of their reproductive life to another. This is a natural part of the life cycle of a woman's body.

The Life Stages of PMS

To understand why a woman's vulnerability to PMS changes through the years, it helps to consider what's happening in her body over the course of her menstrual life. As it happens, there are key times in a woman's life when premenstrual symptoms are likely to flare up or worsen. During the normal transitions of a woman's reproductive life—when she first begins to get her period, in the months after having a baby, and toward the end of her menstrual life, in particular—all sorts of premenstrual symptoms may become more pronounced. In fact, one in five women with severe PMS reports an onset that's associated with her first menstrual period or following childbirth. What's the connection? During these reproductive milestones in a woman's life, there may be an upset in her body's natural state of balance (or homeostasis), or she may experience role overload and/or the stress of adjusting to a new stage of life. In particular, mood symptoms such as anxiety, tension, hyper-reactivity, and anger seem to be especially exaggerated during a woman's adult years, particularly in her thirties. On the other hand, physical symptoms such as breast tenderness, pain, and bloating tend to intensify when a woman first gets her period in adolescence and later in life, prior to menopause.

All of these fluctuations are related to the disregulation of the menstrual cycle, to unpredictable surges of hormones that typically occur at the beginning or end of a woman's reproductive years. This disregulation can be related to the disruption of the body's hormonal balance or to a woman's heightened sensitivity to external stimuli (such as work stress) or internal stimuli (such as changes in levels of neurotransmitters). Regardless of what sparks it, disregulation occurs when various aspects of the menstrual cycle, as well as factors that affect the menstrual cycle, stop working in harmony and start doing their own thing. This can lead to hormonal havoc and unpleasant symptoms.

THE DAWNING OF THE MENSTRUAL AGE

Between the ages of nine and 16, most girls will have entered puberty, which occurs when the ovaries are activated by the brain and begin producing hormones that cause changes in cognition and mood as well as the development of breasts, underarm and pubic hair growth, and gradually the onset of menstruation. The first menstrual period usually occurs once the breasts have begun developing and the body reaches a critical weight and composition. A growth spurt, along with fat and weight gain, usually occurs shortly after a girl's period has begun. Before long, her growth rate will slow considerably and her ultimate height will be achieved. It may, however, take several years for the menstrual cycle to stabilize into a regular pattern.

During adolescence, girls begin to experience the development of a menstrual rhythm and increasing awareness of their own premenstrual and menstrual changes and symptoms. For the most part, research has found that girls who've begun to menstruate have negative evaluations of the monthly cycle, viewing menstruation as debilitating or bothersome. While some feel more grown up now that they're menstruating, others become self-conscious, embarrassed, and secretive about their experiences. In study after study, girls have emphasized the central role their mothers play in their own menstrual experience. Indeed, young women's menstrual and premenstrual experiences are largely shaped by the attitudes of their family members and peers as well as the media. Not only is there a family resemblance in attitudes towards menstruation, but research has found that mothers and daughters tend to resemble each other with respect to symptom experiences as well. Although mothers tend to experience more water retention, there is little difference between them and their offspring on other premenstrual and menstrual symptoms.

In addition, girls often influence each other's premenstrual experiences. In one study, researchers found that shortly after they began to menstruate, young women reported less severe menstrual distress than what girls who hadn't begun to menstruate expected to experience. Because the expectations of these younger girls paralleled the premenstrual changes reported by adults and older adolescent women, the researchers suggested that the socialization process rather than biology may be responsible for their negative expectations about their symptoms. During this time of enormous physical, emotional, personal, and social changes, adolescent girls are struggling to develop their own sense of individuality, their own moral compass, their own way of handling relationships, and their own sense of competency. Because they're often confused about what's happening to their bodies, they often adopt dismal attitudes toward menstruation if that's what they're hearing from their mothers or their friends. This negative mindset can, in turn, increase their vulnerability to PMS through the power of suggestion.

THE WONDROUS REPRODUCTIVE YEARS

The next vulnerable time for the onset or aggravation of PMS is during the postpartum period. During the months after giving birth, a woman may not ovulate regularly, or if she's breast-feeding her child, she may have a slight imbalance between estrogen and progesterone. Depending on how sensitive she is to these hormones—each woman has her own threshold for sensitivity—her symptoms may become more intense than ever before, especially if they're exacerbated by emotional stress. As joyful as it may be to have a baby, the weeks and months following childbirth are filled with change and exhaustion. Between the sleep deprivation, the frequent feedings, the added responsibility of caring for a newborn, and the disruptions to the household's equilibrium, it's hardly surprising that up to 20 percent of new mothers will experience postpartum depression. Those who do may also wind up with more severe PMS. In fact, the latest research suggests that women who have suffered severe postpartum depression may be at an increased risk for the most extreme form of PMS. In my own research, one-third of women with moderately severe PMS experienced postpartum depression for longer than two weeks.

Take Whitney, 37, as an example: During her teen years, she suffered mild acne and cramping before the start of her period but no mood symptoms. After she had a baby at the age of 20, however, she felt depressed for many months. "Even though I wasn't married, I really wanted the baby," she explains. "But after I had him, I felt completely out of control, which I hated. I constantly worried that I wasn't going to be a good mother. I worried about how I was going to support us and go to school. I felt either tired or wired all the time."

Gradually, the dark veil of depression lifted, but Whitney, a hair stylist, was left with a lingering reminder of that difficult time: PMS. After she stopped nursing and her period made its return, she began to experience mood swings, crying jags, irritability, water retention, and low back pain, starting about ten days before the onset of her period. When she consulted a doctor about these cyclical symptoms later, she didn't find a sympathetic ear or relief. And in the intervening years, the mood swings and bloating simply got worse, not better.

The effect can swing the other way, too: If a woman has PMS, she may be more prone to postpartum depression later. In a study at Baylor College of Medicine in Houston, researchers found a 43 percent incidence of postpartum depression in women with severe PMS, compared to a 12 percent incidence in women without PMS. Indeed, the risk factors for postpartum depression are similar to those for PMS: a previous episode of depression, a history of difficult life events, a family history of depression or another psychiatric disorder, and sensitivity to marked hormonal shifts. Whether PMS or postpartum depression comes first, it's as if a woman becomes primed for mood swings to come. It's a most unfortunate double whammy that's due, in all likelihood, to a woman's personal sensitivity to times of hormonal change. In fact, clinical reports from obstetricians and psychiatrists who treat women with postpartum depression suggest that these episodes prepare the brain for the onset of PMS later when stress levels increase or hormonal fluctuations occur. The brain, it seems, has a steel-trap memory.

Even if a woman doesn't have a child, there's a chance that her premenstrual symptoms will worsen in her thirties. Many studies have found that older women report more symptoms premenstrually and younger women report more symptoms during menstruation. No one knows exactly why this is but one factor that is clearly related to age is the proportion of ovulatory and anovulatory cycles. In one study, researchers examined the rates of ovulation in 254 women and found that only 62 percent of women between the ages of 20 and 24 ovulated every cycle compared to 91 percent of women between the ages of 30 and 39. This is significant because women have fewer premenstrual symptoms during naturally induced anovulatory cycles compared to ovulatory cycles. Another theory is that as women age, brain receptors are not as resilient to hormonal fluctuations as they were in their earlier years. This may be one reason why premenstrual mood symptoms often become more pronounced as women approach perimenopause.

THE MENSTRUAL YEARS' FINAL ACT

Years before a woman reaches menopause, which is marked by the one-year anniversary of her last period, she enters a phase called peri-menopause, during which her menstrual cycles become irregular. The median age for perimenopause is 47.5, according to the International Menopause Society, and it lasts an average of four years. Like puberty, this is a phase of life that is characterized by uncertainty, only in this case the unpredictability stems from not knowing when your period will come or go as well as whether or not it will bring bothersome symptoms. (Of course, with the onset of irregular periods, many women find it difficult to predict the arrival of the premenstrual phase, which can also make them feel edgy.) To this day, no one knows what a "normal" perimenopause is: It can last an average of four to five years but it can range from as few as one or two years to the better part of a decade. While some women are symptom-free during this transition, others have physical and mood symptoms that are disabling. And while some women abruptly see their periods end, as if a faucet were quickly turned off, others menstruate erratically for years.

Perimenopause has been described by some women as "a bad case of PMS" but the truth is that premenstrual symptoms can actually inten-sify during the perimenopause even as new symptoms that are related to the menopausal process are emerging. Premenstrual mood changes that were not distressing at an earlier stage of life may now be more severe. Or sleep disturbances that occurred only for a night or two before the arrival of a woman's period may now strike every night for a week or so. In addition, a woman may begin to experience night sweats premenstrually. Despite all these changes, the first true sign of the perimenopausal transition is a change in the length of the menstrual cycle or the flow of the menstrual period. Cycles can become shorter or longer and menstrual flow is likely to increase along with mid-cycle bleeding or spotting.

These changes are rooted in hormonal alterations, particularly at the level of the ovaries. By the time a woman reaches her late thirties, the number of ovarian follicles declines rapidly; by the time she enters her forties, she is probably ovulating less regularly than she used to. As a result, a menstrual cycle may pass without ovulation occurring, which would result in irregular bleeding or no period at all. Or, it may result in the release of two eggs, which may account for the increased rate of twins that are born to women over 40. As ovulation becomes increasingly erratic, so do estrogen and progesterone levels. And in many women, both hormones can drop precipitously as well as reaching high peaks.

Instead of having the two hormones cycle in a modulated rhythm of synchronized harmony, these perimenopausal changes can produce discordant waves of estrogen and progesterone, waves that sputter erratically or peak and crash like a sea in the midst of a violent storm. Scientists believe that these perimenopausal surges and drops in ovarian hormones play a role in a number of menstrual disorders as well as the onset or intensification of perimenopausal and premenstrual symptoms. Many body functions—including sleep, memory, mood, energy, immune action, skin health, and sexual function—are affected by these acute fluctuations. Depending on the intensity of the hormonal fluctuations, a woman's own sensitivity to hormonal changes, and her vulnerability to stress, she may experience one or more of these changes during the perimenopause.

Moreover, during the perimenopause, a woman's typical PMS symptoms may become more intense. By some estimates, 60 to 80 percent of women experience mild to moderate premenstrual symptoms during perimenopause while up to 20 percent of women will experience more severe PMS. A contributing factor could be that stress may be more severe during the perimenopausal transition as women at midlife have to cope with balancing work and family responsibilities that may include both children and aging parents—the stress of the so-called "sandwich generation." In addition, some women may have developed health-harming coping strategies (such as ruminating about their problems or engaging in negative self-talk) or health-damaging habits (such as overeating, being a couch potato, or abusing alcohol) along the way that could exacerbate their premenstrual symptoms. On the other hand, women who have cultivated healthy habits or implemented their own PMS symptom–management plans may find that they experience only mild symptoms at this time.

When Stress Fans the Flames of PMS

Regardless of a woman's age, a number of studies have suggested that either stressful life experiences influence the reporting of premenstrual symptoms or that stressful physical, psychological, and social factors increase the severity of PMS. A study at Queens University in Kingston, Ontario, for example, found that 44 percent of the women with severe PMS continued to report a few negative mood symptoms even after their periods ended, although at a lower severity. This group differed from the other women with severe PMS in that they had significantly more negative life changes—such as marital separation or divorce, or employment changes—in the past year, a tendency to respond to stress with anxiety, and lower scores on measures of self-esteem. It could be that these women had a subclinical anxiety disorder or that the postmenstrual negative mood symptoms were like a PMS hangover, a carryover effect of severe PMS that, in turn, caused long-lasting disruption to their lives.

The similarities between premenstrual symptoms and various aspects of the stress response have prompted some researchers and clinicians to suggest that environmental changes as well as hormonal changes across the menstrual cycle stimulate a neuroendocrine response that results in premenstrual symptoms. Indeed, fluctuations in the severity or experience of PMS are related to a woman's emotional and behavioral responses to these physical events or to other sources of stress in her life. After all, these hormonal shifts don't happen in isolation. They happen in the context of a woman's life, which means that everyday hassles, the stress that's associated with adjusting to new life stages, and the amount of support a woman has (or doesn't) from other people can profoundly affect her experience with PMS or exacerbate her symptoms.

With prolonged stress, which continuously activates the body's fight-or-flight response, the body's natural state of balance, or homeostasis, is disrupted. When the adrenal glands are constantly driven to respond and churn out hormones such as adrenaline, this can upset the balance of other hormones in the body which can trigger headaches, panic attacks, digestive distress, skin problems, and overwhelming fatigue. Then, too, high levels of adrenaline and other stress hormones can aggravate premenstrual symptoms such as mood swings and water retention or lead to premenstrual magnification (PMM) of an underlying condition such as asthma.

Sometimes it's difficult to separate biology from behavior, to distinguish whether a woman's premenstrual symptoms become exaggerated because of her reproductive stage of life or because of her perception of and reaction to her life's circumstances. In my research, I have found that women with moderately severe PMS—regardless of their age and stage of life—do not handle stress well and their emotional reactivity to stress simply increases during the premenstrual phase of their cycles. Upon closer investigation, it became apparent that one-third of these women experienced low self-esteem throughout the menstrual cycle. During the premenstrual phase, however, their feelings of self-esteem and well-being declined, and they often used maladaptive coping strategies such as binge-eating and over-scheduling to take their minds off their distress.

By becoming aware of the stages of life when your vulnerability to premenstrual symptoms is likely to spike, and by becoming aware of how you generally respond to stress, you can become more attuned to physical, emotional, and behavioral changes you're likely to experience in relation to the menstrual cycle. This increased awareness can help you be proactive: If you take steps now to improve your ability to manage stress, enhance your sense of well-being, and clean up your health habits, you may be able to prevent or mitigate some of these flare-ups throughout your reproductive life. Not only will this help you free yourself from the tyranny of hormonal fluctuations, but you'll also be practicing good self-care, which can boost your physical and emotional health in all sorts of ways.

PART TWO

Learning to Manage These Cyclical Shifts

3

Getting in Touch with Your Symptoms

It's the luteal phase of your menstrual cycle: Do you know what your body is trying to tell you? Before considering how to best ease premenstrual symptoms, it's a good idea to pinpoint patterns of symptoms you usually experience, what factors seem to exacerbate them, and when they're likely to flare up. Because the range of symptoms that are associated with PMS is so broad, and because they can also be related to stress or other problems, it's important to identify which ones are particularly troublesome for you and when they are likely to occur in the menstrual cycle. As you know, there's no diagnostic test that will reveal that, yes, indeed, you do have PMS. It's generally diagnosed based on the cyclicity and severity of your symptoms and their reccurrence on a monthly basis just before the arrival of your period.

Tracking your symptoms is the first crucial step in identifying these patterns. Don't be surprised if you discover that some of the symptoms you've been attributing to premenstrual changes actually occur at other times of the month, too. By the same token, you might find that other symptoms you thought were occurring randomly are actually occurring with some degree of predictability premenstrually. Many women reveal such eye-opening connections in the course of charting their symptoms.

After all, symptoms of many conditions can resemble PMS but they're really just great pretenders. All sorts of different conditions can cause fatigue, for example—allergies, anemia, depression, diabetes, heart disease, and thyroid problems, among others—but the key to determining whether PMS is to blame for your fatigue is the timing of the symptoms. Fatigue that is connected to PMS will occur only in the second half of the menstrual cycle, rather than all month long as it would with these other conditions. If your symptoms don't fit a PMS pattern, the self-assessment component of the program will help you and your health-care practitioner determine what the underlying problem may be.

Evaluating your symptoms and discussing them with a health-care professional can also help you distinguish between changes in your ability to function physically, psychologically, or socially and potential signs of an underlying illness or condition. Assessing and monitoring your symptoms can be particularly helpful in this respect: Once you have a record of your premenstrual symptoms over, say, two or three menstrual cycles, you can use these cues as a guide for appropriate treatments to manage these symptoms on your own. And if you decide to seek professional help for some aspect of your premenstrual symptoms—or for premenstrual magnification of an underlying condition—your record can serve as proof to your health-care provider that you are experiencing cyclical flare-ups of symptoms that may require medical attention. Plus, this record will provide your health-care practitioner with highly specific information that will be useful for diagnosis and treatment recommendations.

Research on premenstrual symptoms has found that the mood symptoms (such as irritability or mood swings) and behavioral changes (such as food cravings, or acting or speaking impulsively) are generally the most distressing for women. Here are the five primary ways in which symptoms typically stack up:

Mood-related symptoms can actually be subdivided into two clusters: What I call **Turmoil**, which includes anxiety, nervousness, restlessness, anger or hostility, tension, rapid mood changes, impatience, irritability, oversensitivity, and feeling overwhelmed; and **The Blues**, which includes feeling depressed or sad, crying easily, loneliness, a lowered desire to talk or move, feelings of unattractiveness, low self-image, and sleeping more than usual.

Pain/discomfort symptoms include bloating, swelling in the hands or feet, breast tenderness, abdominal or pelvic pain, headaches, joint aches, backaches, and muscle stiffness.

Somatic/cognitive symptoms include fatigue, constipation, diarrhea, nausea, gas, acne, skin itching, weight gain, forgetfulness, confusion, poor judgment, night sweats, and hot flashes.

Behavioral/functional changes include increased appetite, food cravings, overeating or bingeing (on food or alcohol), feeling out of control, acting impulsively (such as having angry outbursts), poor coordination or clumsiness, distractibility, being disorganized, sleep disturbances, a drop in sexual desire, decreased efficiency, and lowered work performance.

Most women will experience a combination of mood and behavioral changes, along with some physical or cognitive symptoms. If you were to rate the anxiety/anger mood symptoms ("Turmoil") as most distressing, then you are likely to also experience behavioral changes such as feeling out of control, acting or speaking impulsively, increased appetite, overeating or bingeing, and disturbed sleep. If you were to fall into the depressive/withdrawn mood cluster ("The Blues"), on the other hand, you'd be more likely to experience behavioral changes such as social withdrawal, sleeping more than usual, feeling lethargic or tired, and a drop in sexual desire. In other words, the changes in your mood engender changes in your behavior or the way you feel physically.

While some women will have only distressing physical, cognitive, or pain symptoms, many women rate the mood symptoms as most severe or bothersome and some of the pain or discomfort symptoms as less severe. Simply put, the physical symptoms are often secondary to the mood symptoms, at least in the minds of the beholders. Women often find these mood changes scarier or harder to deal with than the physical sensations because the emotional swings can make a woman feel as if she's out of control, losing her mind, or becoming a monster. The mood changes can also be more disruptive to work and family life—and they may last longer than the physical sensations. Hence, they tend to eclipse the physical symptoms on the scale of bothersome complaints. But that doesn't mean premenstrual physical discomfort doesn't deserve attention in its own right. The most common premenstrual pain or discomfort symptoms are breast tenderness, abdominal bloating, and swelling of the hands, ankles, and feet, and women in both the "Turmoil" and "The Blues" mood categories are likely to experience one or more of these symptoms to some degree.

Once you recognize the clusters your primary symptoms fall into, you can tailor your treatment accordingly. If pain, headaches, and bloating are the most bothersome symptoms for you, you might start with dietary changes to prevent those symptoms or ease their severity. If emotional symptoms—mood swings and irritability, for example— are the biggest offenders, you might focus your energy on identifying and modifying the primary sources of stress in your work or personal life and employing breathing techniques or other relaxation exercises to help you calm down.

Assessing Your Symptoms, Yourself

Getting in touch with your symptoms means more than simply listing and rating your feelings, symptoms, and behavioral changes. It involves cultivating self-awareness and initiating a process of self-monitoring that includes a focus on both you and your environment—your scheduling practices, your physical surroundings, and the people in your life. After all, premenstrual changes don't occur in a vacuum. They occur in the context of your life so they need to be examined accordingly. In later chapters, you will learn how to evaluate your dietary and nutritional practices, your physical activity and exercise habits, your life stress and relationship pressures to see how they affect your premenstrual experience.

Before we go any further, we want to introduce the "PMS Notebook" as a tool for creating your personalized PMS plan. Because of all the factors that are used to custom-tailor your PMS plan, we recommend that you develop a notebook to organize the various forms and charts that you will find in the upcoming chapters as well as the appendix. In my research, women found that using a three-ring binder with dividers—corresponding to sections on history, symptom tracking, symptom management strategies, and personal notes—was highly useful. You can either write in this book or make copies of selected pages and charts to add to your notebook.

This Is Your (Menstrual) Life

First, though, it's time to look back at your life and take stock of your past and current health status. If you wind up seeking professional advice, this information will be invaluable because it will succinctly provide your health and menstrual history. Set aside some free time to do your homework, take out a pad of paper and a pen, and answer the following questions. Or, you may want to copy these pages, place them in your notebook, and answer the questions there. That way, if you wind up needing to consult a health professional, data on your medical, health, and PMS history will be at your fingertips.

- In your own words, describe the premenstrual symptoms that are the most severe or distressing to you.

- What is the pattern of symptoms during a typical menstrual cycle? How many days before or after your period do you notice these symptoms? Do they occur around ovulation?

- Does anything in particular—work stress, dietary influences, or exercise, for example—worsen or alleviate your symptoms?

- How old were you when PMS first began?

- Did the onset coincide with a specific event such as your first period, following childbirth, or the use of birth control pills, for instance?

- Do you generally have the same symptoms every cycle? Is the severity the same each month?

- Do you notice that you are more easily affected by alcohol premenstrually?

- Do you notice marked fluctuations in your weight at different times of the cycle?

- Do your mother or sister(s) have PMS or did they ever?

- How many days of work have you missed in the last three months because of PMS?

- If you have not missed work, how many days in the last three months has your work efficiency or productivity been affected? Has a supervisor or a colleague noticed this change?

- What are the negative effects of PMS on your life?

- Can you describe any positive feelings or changes that are associated with menstruation or the menstrual cycle?

- Do you have regular menstrual cycles (meaning the number of days between periods is usually the same)?

- How many days are there from the start of one period to the start of the next?

- How old were you when you first started to menstruate?

- Have you experienced any changes in your menstrual cycle since you began getting your period?

- Have you experienced an adverse reaction to oral contraceptives or symptoms associated with sterilization?

- Have you experienced postpartum symptoms for more than two weeks after giving birth? Have you ever received professional treatment for postpartum depression?

- Did you experience PMS-like symptoms during pregnancy?

- Do you notice any variations in chronic conditions—such as allergies, asthma, arthritis, migraines, skin conditions, depression, fibroids, endometriosis, or vulvovaginitis—that seem to be related to where you are in the menstrual cycle?

Next, spend a few minutes evaluating your personal status and lifestyle habits in the following areas:

DIET AND NUTRITION

- How do you rate your overall diet on a scale of zero (unhealthy) to ten (very healthy)?

- How do you perceive your weight: as underweight, normal weight, or overweight?

- What vitamins and minerals do you take on a regular basis?

- What other nutritional supplements do you take?

- Do you crave alcohol or certain foods? Which foods or tastes do you crave?

- Do you binge on food or alcohol? Does it happen at certain times of the day or menstrual cycle?

- How often do you binge?

- To what extent does food control your life?

PHYSICAL ACTIVITY

- How would you describe your level of physical activity (from couch potato to weekend warrior to consistently active)?

- How much exercise do you get in an average week?

- What types of exercise do you perform consistently?

- What types of physical activities do you perform occasionally?

SLEEP

- How well rested do you generally feel?

- How many hours of sleep do you get each night?

- What time do you usually go to bed? How long does it take for you to fall asleep?

- During the night do you have any problems with staying asleep or early morning awakening?

- What time do you usually wake up?

- Do you take naps?

- Do you use sleep medications or aids?

STRESS

- How would you characterize your general stress level over the last three months on a scale of zero to ten (with zero being none and ten being extreme)?

- How stressful is your work, again on a scale of zero to ten?

- How stressful are your relationships within your immediate family (zero to ten)?

- How stressful is your relationship with your spouse or intimate partner (zero to ten)?

- How emotionally taxing are your close friendships (zero to ten)?

- How stressful is your relationship with your children or your feelings about parenting (zero to ten)?

WELL-BEING

- How would you characterize your general level of well-being over the last three months on a scale of zero to ten (with zero being none and ten being very high)?

- You can also rate your feelings of well-being as they relate to different aspects of your life—work, family, romance/intimacy, children, friends, and so on.

Your Premenstrual Checklists

Now that you've had a chance to look back at your overall health history, it's time to take a closer look at your patterns of premenstrual symptoms. Think about your premenstrual experiences over the last three to six months and consider which symptoms, in particular, have bothered you most consistently. Does your premenstrual discomfort cluster into a group that looks like one of the following five patterns during the week or so before your period? Or do you have some symptoms from each category? To find out, circle all the symptoms that occur most regularly in the second half of your menstrual cycle then see where the majority reside.

The benefit to performing this exercise is that you'll be able to tell whether your symptoms reside in a particular cluster or whether they're all over the map. Most women don't think about whether their depressive symptoms ("The Blues") are more dominant than their turmoil symptoms or vice versa, for example. Nor do they consider

The Cluster Checklist

INSTRUCTIONS: *Circle the symptoms or behavior changes that are most bothersome to you before or during your period.*

Mood

TURMOIL SYMPTOMS

Anger or hostility

Irritability

Anxiety

Nervousness

Restlessness, feeling jittery

Tension

Rapid mood changes

Impatience

Over-sensitivity

Feeling overwhelmed

THE BLUES SYMPTOMS

Feeling depressed or blue

Crying easily

Feeling lonely

Low self-image

Lowered desire to talk or move

Less interest in usual activities

Thoughts of self-harm

Pain/Discomfort

Abdominal bloating

Swelling in hands, feet

Headaches

Pelvic cramps

Breast tenderness

Back- or neckaches

Body aches and pains

Muscle stiffness

Joint pain

Behavioral/Functional Changes

Food cravings

Increased appetite

Alcohol cravings

Overeating or bingeing—food or alcohol

Feeling out of control

Acting, speaking impulsively

Sleep disturbances

Lowered work performance

Decreased efficiency

Disorganized (more than usual)

Clumsiness

Poor coordination

Distractibility

Social withdrawal

Drop in sexual desire

Sleeping excessively

Somatic/Cognitive

Constipation

Diarrhea

Indigestion

Nausea

Acne

Skin itching

Weight gain

Fatigue

Forgetfulness

Confusion

Poor judgment

Night sweats

Hot flashes

Dizziness

Heart palpitations

whether they're more bothered by physical symptoms or feelings or behaviors during the premenstrual phase. This checklist will help you tease out these distinctions. You'll also be able to see how many symptoms you typically experience, which is significant because there's a high correlation between the number of symptoms and the severity of PMS. Ultimately, this newfound knowledge will be useful in helping you figure out how to start your treatment.

The Premenstrual Symptom Severity Chart

Once you have a pulse on your premenstrual symptom patterns and their effects on your life, it's wise to examine the severity of your symptoms. Again, reflect back on the last three to six months and consider how you typically felt during the week or two before each period as well as during the first three days of your period. Then, use the Premenstrual Symptom Severity Chart to gauge the intensity of your symptoms in the latter half of your menstrual cycle. If you have had a recurring symptom or experience that is not included on this list, write it in the "other" space and rate it accordingly.

The Premenstrual Symptom Severity Chart

SYMPTOM SEVERITY RATING SYSTEM

0 = Absent or None

1 = Mild	*"I notice the feeling, symptom, or behavior but it doesn't interfere with activities or make me feel distressed."*
2 = Moderate	*"This symptom affects my work, the way I feel, or my ability to function but even though I feel somewhat distressed, I'm able to carry on with my usual activities."*
3 = Severe	*"This symptom limits or interferes with my activities; I feel distressed that I can't do what I want to do.*
4 = Extreme	*"I feel very distressed by the feeling, symptom, or behavior; I can't do anything; I stay in bed or don't get dressed."*

INSTRUCTIONS: *Rate each feeling, symptom, or behavior change on this 0 to 4 scale that best describes how you feel before or during your period.*

1. Abdominal bloating 0   1   2   3   4
2. Acting, speaking impulsively 0   1   2   3   4
3. Alcohol cravings 0   1   2   3   4
4. Anger 0   1   2   3   4
5. Anxiety 0   1   2   3   4

6. Backache or neckache 0   1   2   3   4
7. Constipation 0   1   2   3   4
8. Clumsiness 0   1   2   3   4
9. Decreased efficiency 0   1   2   3   4
10. Depression/felt sad or blue 0   1   2   3   4

11. Diarrhea 0   1   2   3   4
12. Difficulty concentrating 0   1   2   3   4
13. Difficulty falling asleep 0   1   2   3   4
14. Disorganized (more than usual) 0   1   2   3   4
15. Distractibility 0   1   2   3   4

16. Fatigue or tiredness 0   1   2   3   4
17. Feeling unattractive .0   1   2   3   4
18. Food cravings 0   1   2   3   4
19. Forgetfulness 0   1   2   3   4
20. Generalized body aches 0   1   2   3   4

21. Headache 0   1   2   3   4
22. Hot flashes/sudden flushes of warmth 0   1   2   3   4
23. Hostility 0   1   2   3   4
24. Impatience 0   1   2   3   4
25. Indigestion/upset stomach 0   1   2   3   4

26. Irritability 0   1   2   3   4
27. Joint pain or stiffness 0   1   2   3   4
28. Loneliness 0   1   2   3   4
29. Loss of appetite 0   1   2   3   4
30. Loss of interest in things 0   1   2   3   4

31. Loss of sexual interest 0   1   2   3   4
32. Lowered desire to talk or move 0   1   2   3   4
33. Lowered work performance 0   1   2   3   4
34. Nausea 0   1   2   3   4
35. Nervousness, feeling jittery 0   1   2   3   4

36. Night sweats 0   1   2   3   4
37. Mood swings 0   1   2   3   4
38. Out of control feelings 0   1   2   3   4
39. Overeating, bingeing on food/alcohol 0   1   2   3   4
40. Overwhelmed 0   1   2   3   4

41. Over-sensitivity 0   1   2   3   4
42. Painful or tender breasts 0   1   2   3   4
43. Panicky feelings 0   1   2   3   4
44. Poor coordination 0   1   2   3   4
45. Poor judgment 0   1   2   3   4

46. Restlessness 0   1   2   3   4
47. Skin breakout/acne .0   1   2   3   4
48. Skin itching 0   1   2   3   4
49. Sleeping too much .0   1   2   3   4
50. Swelling of hands or feet 0   1   2   3   4

51. Tearfulness/crying spells	....	0	1	2	3	4
52. Tension	....	0	1	2	3	4
53. Thoughts of self-harm	....	0	1	2	3	4
54. Waking up during the night	....	0	1	2	3	4
55. Waking too early	....	0	1	2	3	4
56. Weight gain	....	0	1	2	3	4
57. Withdrawal, avoiding social activities	....	0	1	2	3	4
58. Other	....	0	1	2	3	4
59. Other	....	0	1	2	3	4
60. Other	....	0	1	2	3	4

After completing this evaluation, you will have gained insight into how your symptoms affect the context of your life, where to focus your attention, and what measures to start with in your treatment plan. If you find that pain symptoms are the most bothersome, for example, you might need to start with a basic PMS plan (from Chapter Ten) but you may want to add other interventions that target pain more quickly. This is all a part of setting the stage for custom-tailoring your intervention plan. This evaluative process is quite similar to what health-care practitioners would go through in order to make a medical diagnosis. The difference is, this time the process is in your hands. After all, no one is giving you a prescription for PMS relief. By filling out these evaluation forms, you'll be arming yourself with information that will be meaningful in coming up with your own solution for managing PMS.

The PMS Tracking Chart

When you truly know what you're dealing with, you'll be in a much better position to keep tabs on your symptoms and to determine which treatments may be helping. Much to their surprise, many women discover that self-monitoring their symptoms is an effective treatment by itself because it puts them back in touch with their bodies, instead of remaining at odds with them. In my research, I have found that for up to 15 percent of women, tracking symptoms was enough to reduce the severity of their PMS because they came to see these changes in a more realistic light—they realized they only had a few days of severe symptoms, for example. Others were able to move quickly into making small alterations to their lifestyles, or they may have sought treatment more promptly for menstrual migraines, for instance, if they realized that's what they were dealing with rather than a whole constellation of symptoms.

At this point, you're ready to move forward and carefully monitor your daily symptoms, using the PMS Tracking Chart featured on the next few pages. We've included a completed chart as an example.

The blank chart has horizontal columns for the days of your menstrual cycle and vertical rows with spaces for your symptoms. You'll want to use this chart for at least one month—and maybe two, depending on how regular your cycles are and how quickly you want to move into your treatment plan—as a baseline assessment of what's really happening with your menstrual cycle. Once you've completed a chart of an entire cycle, it will give you an unvarnished look at what's truly going on with your symptoms across the menstrual cycle. Take a close look at your pattern of symptoms: During which phase of the menstrual cycle do you have the most severe symptoms (menstrual, post-menstrual, or premenstrual)? How much variability is there in your symptoms across these phases?

Because PMS has no clearly defined cause, it is important to distinctly delineate your symptoms, their patterns, and how they are related (or not) to your menstrual cycle. You might find, for example, that your mood or behavior changes—which may have been heightened during the premenstrual phase—were actually due to external problems such as work-related stress, relationship difficulties, problems with kids, or other legitimate sources of anxiety, fear, and frustration. Alternatively, when examining your completed chart, you might discover that you have some physical symptoms that you don't like—acne or bloating, for example—but that these really aren't a big deal because they last for only a couple of days. Overall, this exercise will help you gain a sense of self-awareness and become more attuned to how your premenstrual symptoms manifest themselves as symptoms, feelings, or behaviors, as well as the degree to which they affect your life.

CHART 3.3

PMS Tracking Chart

Menstrual Cycle Day	1	2	3	4	5	6	7	8	9	10	11	12	13
Month __Sept/Oct__ Date	9/25	26	27	28	29	30	10/1	2	3	4	5	6	7
Menstrual Cycle Phase	Menstrual Phase					↑	PostMenstrual Phase						
Bleeding (H, M, L, S, *)	S	H	H	M	L	*							
Weight	135		134		133								
SYMPTOMS (0–4)													
1. Irritability	3	1	0	0	0	0	0	0	0	0	0	0	0
2. Anxiety	4	2	0	0	0	0	0	0	0	0	0	0	0
3. Over-sensitive	3	2	0	0	0	0	0	0	0	0	0	0	0
4. Cry easily	3	1	0	0	0	0	0	0	0	0	0	0	0
5. Out of control	4	2	0	0	0	0	0	0	0	0	0	0	0
6. Act out	3	1	0	0	0	0	0	0	0	0	0	0	0
7. Bloating	4	3	2	1	0	0	0	0	0	0	0	0	0
8. Swelling	3	3	1	0	0	0	0	0	0	0	0	0	0
9. Difficulty falling asleep	3	1	1	0	0	0	0	0	0	0	0	0	0
10. Confusion	2	2	0	0	0	0	0	0	0	0	0	0	0
Well-being (+ / –)	/	/	+	+	+	+	+	/	/	+	+	+	+
Stress (+ / –)	/	/	/	–	–	–	–	/	/	–	–	–	–
Life Events (+ / –)	/	/	/	+	+	/	/	/	+	+	/	/	/
SELF-CARE													
1. Left work/stay home	√												
2. Take a walk	√	√											
3. Call my friend		√											

TRACKING INSTRUCTIONS:

1. **Menstrual Cycle Day:** Begin with the first day of menstrual flow and end with the last day of your menstrual cycle.

2. **Month and Date:** Write in the month then the corresponding date in the box under each menstrual cycle day.

3. **Menstrual Cycle Phase:** At the end of the cycle, divide it into phases by drawing a vertical line down after the day before menstrual bleeding starts; count back 14 days, draw another vertical line, and write *premenstrual phase* in the space; next, draw a vertical line down after the last day of your period and write in *menstrual* phase; write in *postmenstrual phase* in the remaining space.

4. **Bleeding:** Record your menstrual flow or vaginal bleeding as (H) Heavy, (M) Moderate, (L) Light, (S) Spotting, or blank if no bleeding. Note the last day of your menstrual flow with an asterisk (*).

14	15	16	17	18	19	20	21	22	23	24	25	26	27	28	29	30	31	32
8	9	10	11	12	13	14	15	16	17	18	19	20	21	22	23			
↑						Pre-Menstrual Phase									↑			
																S		
133											133		134		135			
0	0	1	1	1	1	2	2	2	2	3	3	4	4	4	3			
0	0	1	2	2	2	2	2	2	2	2	2	3	3	3	3			
0	0	1	2	2	2	2	2	2	2	3	3	3	3	3	3			
0	0	0	0	0	0	0	0	1	1	2	2	2	2	3	3			
0	0	1	1	1	2	2	2	2	2	2	3	3	3	3	3			
0	0	0	0	1	1	2	2	1	1	2	2	2	3	3	3			
0	0	0	0	0	0	0	0	1	2	2	2	3	4	4	4			
0	0	0	0	0	0	0	0	1	2	2	2	3	3	3	3			
1	1	0	0	1	1	1	0	1	2	2	2	2	3	2	3			
0	0	0	0	0	0	0	0	0	0	0	0	0	0	2	2			
+	+	+	/	/	/	/	/	/	/	–	–	–	–	–	–			
–	–	–	–	–	–	+	+	+	+	+	/	/	+	/	+			
/	/	/	/	/	/	+	/	/	/	/	/	/	/	/	/			
														√				
												√	√	√				
										√		√			√			

5. **Weight:** Record your weight (weigh yourself about the same time every day).

6. **Symptoms:** List your most bothersome or distressing symptoms taken from the Symptom Severity Chart with your worst or most distressing symptom in the #1 space, followed by your second most bothersome symptom, and so on, up to 10 symptoms. Rate these symptoms or behavior changes daily as 0-absent, 1-mild, 2-moderate, 3-severe, or 4-extreme throughout the cycle.

7. **Well-being:** Rate your feelings of well-being—including increased energy, creativity, or generally feeling good—as (+) High, (/) Moderate, or (–) Low.

8. **Stress:** Rate your overall stress level as (+) High, (/) Moderate, or (–) Low.

9. **Life Events:** Rate any significant events as (+) Positive, (/) Neutral, or (–) Negative.

10. **Self-Care:** List anything you did to relieve your symptoms and place a check in the corresponding menstrual day.

PMS Tracking Chart

Menstrual Cycle Day	1	2	3	4	5	6	7	8	9	10	11	12	13
Month_____ Date													
Menstrual Cycle Phase													
Bleeding (H, M, L, S, *)													
Weight													
SYMPTOMS (0 – 4)													
1.													
2.													
3.													
4.													
5.													
6.													
7.													
8.													
9.													
10.													
Well-being (+ / −)													
Stress (+ / −)													
Life Events (+ / −)													
SELF-CARE													
1.													
2.													
3.													

TRACKING INSTRUCTIONS:

1. **Menstrual Cycle Day:** Begin with the first day of menstrual flow and end with the last day of your menstrual cycle.

2. **Month and Date:** Write in the month then the corresponding date in the box under each menstrual cycle day.

3. **Menstrual Cycle Phase:** At the end of the cycle, divide it into phases by drawing a vertical line down after the day before menstrual bleeding starts; count back 14 days, draw another vertical line, and write *premenstrual phase* in the space; next, draw a vertical line down after the last day of your period and write in *menstrual* phase; write in *postmenstrual phase* in the remaining space.

4. **Bleeding:** Record your menstrual flow or vaginal bleeding as (H) Heavy, (M) Moderate, (L) Light, (S) Spotting, or blank if no bleeding. Note the last day of your menstrual flow with an asterisk (*).

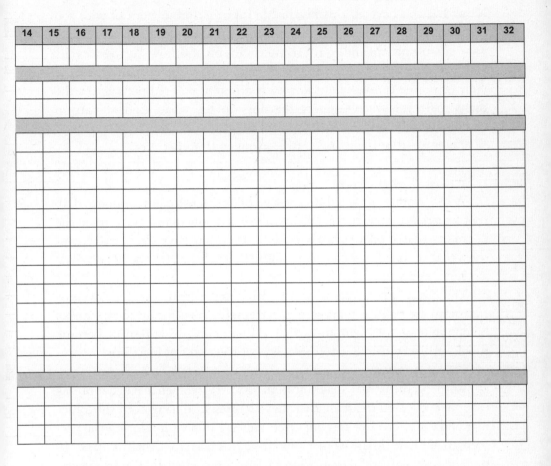

5. **Weight:** Record your weight (weigh yourself about the same time every day).

6. **Symptoms:** List your most bothersome or distressing symptoms taken from the Symptom Severity Chart with your worst or most distressing symptom in the #1 space, followed by your second most bothersome symptom, and so on, up to 10 symptoms. Rate these symptoms or behavior changes daily as 0-absent, 1-mild, 2-moderate, 3-severe, or 4-extreme throughout the cycle.

7. **Well-being:** Rate your feelings of well-being—including increased energy, creativity, or generally feeling good—as (+) High, (/) Moderate, or (–) Low.

8. **Stress:** Rate your overall stress level as (+) High, (/) Moderate, or (–) Low.

9. **Life Events:** Rate any significant events as (+) Positive, (/) Neutral, or (–) Negative.

10. **Self-Care:** List anything you did to relieve your symptoms and place a check in the corresponding menstrual day.

The Best of Times/Worst of Times Graph

Now that you have all this invaluable information in front of you, you can classify your own symptom patterns on a graph to see how severe your symptoms are and to illustrate their ebb and flow during a cycle. Using the grid that's provided on page (54) plot the ups and downs of your top three to five symptoms with different colored pens across the menstrual cycle then connect the dots to see what kind of pattern emerges.

There are three primary classifications of PMS patterns:

1. *Low Severity Pattern*

When women have a low severity of premenstrual symptoms (LS), they experience a few bothersome symptoms of low to mild severity in the postmenstrual or premenstrual phases or they may have one or two symptoms that are rated as moderate to severe but only last for one or two days.

2. *PMS Pattern*

The classic premenstrual syndrome pattern (PMS) includes symptoms that are rated as moderate to extremely severe for up to two weeks before your period, symptoms that subsequently disappear or become much milder within one to three days of the onset of bleeding.

3. *PMM Pattern*

With premenstrual magnification (PMM), women have symptoms that are cyclical in the sense that they are present during both the follicular and early luteal phases but often increase in severity during the premenstrual phase. Many women who have this pattern identify with PMS but they deserve careful evaluation to determine whether they are experiencing a premenstrual exacerbation of another disorder such as depression, anxiety, headaches, allergies, asthma, or irritable bowel syndrome.

Here are Graphics showing the three types of patterns:

Best of Times/Worst of Times Graph: Low Severity (LS) Pattern

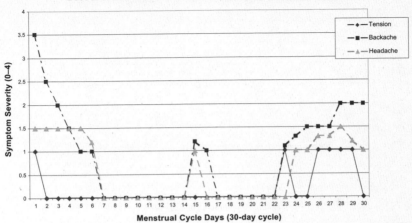

Low Severity (LS) Pattern: Two pain/discomfort symptoms, backache and headache, predominate here but are moderately severe for about 5 to 6 days, mostly during the menstrual phase, dropping to no severity for a week postmenstrually and increasing for 1 to 2 days at ovulation (day 14–16) then again premenstrually (day 22 to onset of next menses on day 30). However, the headache pain is mostly mild and is described as a "tension headache" and the backache is more severe during the woman's period (associated with heavy flow) and mostly mildly severe premenstrually. Negative mood is described as tension and impatience and never increases beyond mild intensity for 6 to 7 days premenstrually.

Best of Times/Worst of Times Graph: PMS Turmoil Pattern

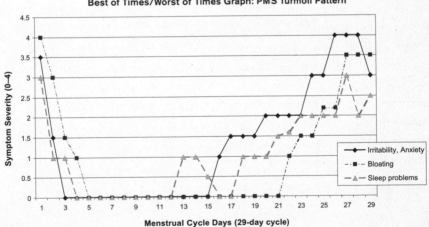

PMS Pattern: Mood symptoms are in the Turmoil cluster with irritability, anxiety, and feeling oversensitive to stress predominating. Feeling out of control and acting impulsively (angry outbursts) followed the same pattern as the mood symptoms. Both mood and behavioral changes increased in severity shortly after midcycle and dropped to zero by the second or third day of the woman's period. Sleep problems included difficulty falling asleep—couldn't put worries out of her mind—and they began about midcycle but increased in severity 5 to 7 days premenstrually. Abdominal bloating and swelling of the feet and ankles were severe to extreme for 4 to 5 days and moderately severe for another 3 to 5 days premenstrually. This PMS pattern is clearly marked with a low severity or symptom-free phase of about 12 to 14 days each month.

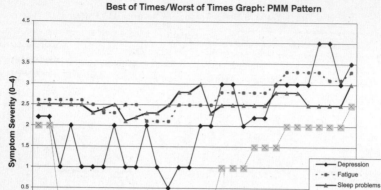

Best of Times/Worst of Times Graph: PMM Pattern

Menstrual Cycle Days (30-day cycle)

PMM Pattern: Mood Symptoms: Depressive feelings, sadness, and feeling lonely would hover between mild to moderate postmenstrually; drop to minimal or mild for a few days around ovulation then gradually increase to severe or extreme premenstrually. Because the depressive symptoms increased along with breast tenderness, she assumed that she had PMS. Sleep problems were a combination of waking up too early and sleeping too much and did not show much of a cyclical pattern. Fatigue and lethargy were related to sleep problems in the postmenstrual phase and increased slightly in severity during the premenstrual phase along with the depressive feelings. Except for breast tenderness, all symptoms were experienced daily across the menstrual cycle; there was no symptom-free phase for the depressive feelings nor for fatigue, lethargy, or sleep.

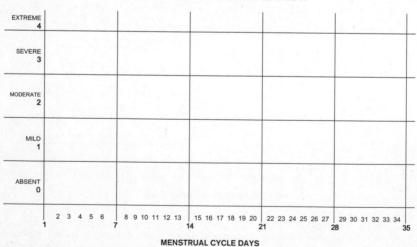

BEST OF TIMES/WORST OF TIMES GRAPH

MENSTRUAL CYCLE DAYS

INSTRUCTIONS:

Plot your worst symptoms: Track the severity of your three to five most bothersome symptoms across one menstrual cycle by transferring the ratings from your PMS Tracking Chart. Plot each day's severity score with a different colored pen using the 0 to 4 severity scale shown on the left vertical axis.

A Snapshot of Your Premenstrual Experience

Review the charts you've filled out so far and transfer the information you now know below. This section will serve as a summary or cheat-sheet to help guide your treatment choices.

YOUR PMS MOOD TYPE

Turmoil   The Blues   Both

YOUR PMS SEVERITY

List your five most bothersome symptoms—those that warranted a rating of 3 (severe) or 4 (extreme):

1. _____

2. _____

3. _____

4. _____

5. _____

THE IMPACT OF PMS ON YOUR LIFE

- How long have you been experiencing PMS—for less than one year, for one to three years, or for more than three years?

  _____

- Would you rate the effect of PMS on your life, including your close, personal relationships, as low, medium, or high?

  _____

- Would you rate the effect of PMS on your work, including your professional relationships, as low, medium, or high?

  _____

- How many days each month do you rate your stress level with a + (indicating high stress)?

  _____

- Is your stress level higher during your premenstrual phase or during your postmenstrual phase?

  _____

- How many days each month do you rate your well-being with a +?

  _____

- Do these feelings change across the menstrual cycle?

  _____

YOUR PMS PATTERN

After rating your symptoms across the menstrual cycle for one month, choose the pattern that most closely describes your experience:

LS
PMS
PMM

If you find after charting and graphing your symptoms that the severity pattern is very erratic across the month or that the symptoms are high all month long (but perhaps higher during the premenstrual phase) or that they peak at a time other than the premenstrual phase (during the postmenstrual phase, for example), you may have more going on than PMS. Your symptoms could be related to stress, a dual diagnosis, a hormonal imbalance, or premenstrual magnification (PMM) of an underlying condition. In that case, read Chapter Thirteen, "Complicating Conditions," and schedule a physical exam with your health-care practitioner. Bring your charts with you. In the meantime, you can't go wrong by starting the PMS management plan because it can help you enhance your health and well-being all month long.

On the other hand, if your symptoms' peaks and valleys do fit neatly into a PMS pattern—meaning, they act up during the week or two before your period and practically disappear within three days of the onset of bleeding—then you'll be able to tailor your treatment accordingly after reading the following chapters of this book. By now, you've probably pinpointed how your mood is typically affected by the premenstrual changes your body experiences each month. You've probably begun to set priorities for the symptoms you'd like to relieve sooner rather than later. And you've probably noticed some basic connections between what's happening in your life and when your premenstrual symptoms tend to ease or worsen. All of this budding self-awareness will help you identify a logical starting point for creating your personalized PMS solution.

4

The PMS Diet

Believe it or not, everything you put in your mouth—from foods to beverages, from vitamins to other nutritional supplements—can have an impact on premenstrual symptoms. In fact, research has found that women with PMS have poorer diets compared to women who don't experience the syndrome. In particular, those with PMS consume three times more refined carbohydrates and simple sugars, more meat and caffeine, and diets that are lower in the B vitamins, iron, zinc, and magnesium. Whether these shabby eating habits cause PMS symptoms or vice versa is a bit of a chicken-and-egg question. But poor food choices certainly don't help these cyclical symptoms. For example, PMS severity, particularly when it comes to irritability and insomnia, is associated with caffeine consumption: Those who drank one caffeine-containing beverage per day experienced symptoms that were 30 percent more intense than those who shirked caffeine; meanwhile, those who drank eight to ten cups of coffee (or its caffeine equivalent per day) had a seven-fold increase in symptom severity, according to a study at Oregon State University.

Your eating habits can have such a sweeping effect on premenstrual symptoms because during the premenstrual phase, many women's bodies are especially sensitive to various stimuli, including the food that enters their bodies. Skipping meals, eating highly processed foods or foods that are high in sugar, or trying to pump yourself up with caffeine, nicotine, or herbal stimulants all can activate the autonomic nervous system, which cracks the whip upon the adrenal glands and other systems, causing more and more stress hormones such as adrenaline, cortisol, and DHEA (dehydroepiandrosterone) to be produced. These changes can, in turn, affect blood-sugar levels, as well as how a woman feels. When these stress hormones flow into the bloodstream in increasing amounts, she may feel agitated, anxious, or otherwise ill at ease. What's more, consuming lots of salty foods and overeating in general can create an imbalance between electrolytes and water in the body, causing abdominal bloating and swelling of the hands, feet, and ankles.

But the domino effect between your eating habits and premenstrual symptoms can fall the other way, too: Many women crave certain types of foods—such as chocolate or salty foods—while they're premenstrual. Your premenstrual symptoms can also affect your dietary behavior because the hormones that regulate the menstrual cycle affect more than just the uterus and the ovaries. Because the menstrual cycle sparks continuous changes in physical and psychological functions, as well as behavior, these cyclical fluctuations can affect a woman's metabolism, her insulin tolerance, her appetite and propensity for food cravings, her mood, and, hence, her eating behavior. Nevertheless, because of the complex nature of eating habits, and the highly individual variation in eating behaviors, it's difficult to draw hard-and-fast conclusions about the effects of menstrual cycle hormones on appetite, hunger, food intake, taste, and food cravings. What we do know from the work of David Rubinow, M.D., at the National Institute of Mental Health, is that estrogen may work to suppress appetite in some way while progesterone may stimulate appetite during the premenstrual phase. One theory is that estrogen lowers dopamine levels which, in turn, decreases brain levels of norepinephrine, a neurotransmitter that is believed to stimulate appetite.

We also know that blood glucose levels rise steadily throughout the menstrual cycle until five to ten days before the onset of a woman's period when they begin to decline; it's possible that this natural decline in blood glucose could be partly responsible for premenstrual carbohydrate cravings (e.g., french fries, chips, cookies, and the like). It may be that during the premenstrual phase of the cycle women are more physiologically sensitive to some of the alterations in blood sugar stability and insulin resistance, as well as to certain foods. Compounding matters, women also may be more vulnerable to these effects due to the physiologic effects of stress—whether it's the stress of PMS or a heightened perception and experience of external sources of stress—on blood sugar, metabolism, and fluid and electrolyte balances.

When you consider these myriad effects, it's no wonder the menstrual cycle's influence on your eating habits can be so powerful. Research has found that all menstruating women seem to have an increased appetite during the last half of the menstrual cycle, perhaps because during the luteal phase the body has a heat-producing response to increased progesterone levels. Because of this heat-producing response, the body burns more calories than usual—an additional 100 to 300 calories a day—but most women naturally eat more during those days, which explains why we don't wind up gaining or losing weight every month.

Interestingly, women with PMS seem to experience a greater increase in appetite and a heightened hunger that lasts for longer than women who don't have PMS. In a study examining the effects of nutrient intake on premenstrual depression, Judith Wurtman, Ph.D., a research scientist at the Massachusetts Institute of Technology, found that women with PMS consumed significantly more food during the premenstrual phase of their cycles: Their energy intake increased from 1,892 calories to 2,395 calories, and their carbohydrate intake jumped 24 percent during meals and 43 percent from snacks.

Nancy, a 43-year-old medical coordinator, is an example of these cyclical swings in eating. Though she constantly worried about her weight and she even joined Weight Watchers, nearly every month her willpower would fly out the window. "For a few days before my period, I'd lose all self-control and binge on sweets," she recalls. "I'd come home from work, eat dinner, and keep eating into the evening. Some nights I could go through a whole bag of cookies or a pint of ice cream. My cravings were so powerful that I couldn't control them."

The trouble is, if you overindulge in sweets, you may experience ups and downs in blood sugar that can leave you feeling drained of energy, or, you could experience even more food cravings than usual, either because your blood sugar is unstable or because you are especially sensitive to the blood sugar swings. If you eat too much salty junk food or highly processed food during the period just before your period, you might feel unusually bloated or wind up with a debilitating headache. Of course, it's not clear if a woman's poor eating habits may be causing her premenstrual symptoms or if her premenstrual food cravings are triggering her poor food choices. Whatever sets this synergistic effect into motion, it's likely to create a continuous cycle of unpleasant symptoms and cravings.

In my own research, more than 55 percent of the women with PMS reported premenstrual food cravings. In addition, one-third of the women with PMS confessed that they sometimes binged and 10 percent did frequently. Not surprisingly, the majority of the women reported that the quality of their dietary habits declined premenstrually.

While there is little scientific evidence that dietary changes alone can eliminate PMS, women who modify their diets during the second half of the menstrual cycle often report substantial improvements in their symptoms. Approximately 90 percent of the women in my own research made changes to their diets, as part of the PMS Symptom Management Program. At first, these modifications were made on an occasional basis, most commonly during the premenstrual phase of their menstrual cycles, but over the long-term, the majority of these women made these practices part of their daily habits. Among the symptoms that were helped the most were irritability, fatigue, anxiety, bloating, and food cravings.

It may not be easy to revamp your eating habits—as any woman who has tried to lose weight well knows—but it can make a considerable difference in how you feel and function, perhaps for as much as half of each month. Your best bet is to tackle these dietary changes in a step-by-step fashion. Fortunately, the dietary guidelines for managing PMS are in sync with the fundamental nutritional recommendations for a healthy body and mind: a low intake of fat and salt, plenty of whole-grain complex carbohydrates, and moderate consumption of caffeine and alcohol. What follows are the key strategies that can make a difference.

GET SAVVY ABOUT SUPPLEMENTS

The first thing I recommend women with PMS do is follow a regimen of vitamin and mineral supplements. These include a general multivitamin with mineral supplement that is taken for half the month (postmenstrually) and a PMS formula supplement (which is specifically for PMS and is found in drugstores) that is taken during the premenstrual phase of your cycle. In my research, half of the women who started their treatment plan with supplements experienced some relief in physical symptoms within the first month and 90 percent continued taking them over the next 18 months.

How can vitamins and minerals help ease PMS symptoms? Vitamin B-6 plays an important role in regulating mood swings, irritability, fatigue, sugar cravings, and fluid retention. Magnesium helps to keep blood sugar levels and mood on a more even keel. Meanwhile, research has found that approximately 40 percent of adults diagnosed with depression have low blood levels of folic acid. And a major study at St. Luke's-Roosevelt Hospital Center in New York City found that calcium supplements eased PMS symptoms such as mood swings, aches and pains, food cravings, and bloating by nearly 50 percent by the third cycle. In my research, PMS-formula vitamin and mineral supplements were the most frequently used strategy and helped to relieve PMS severity—particularly fluid retention, constipation, concentration problems, and mood swings—within the first three months for most women; this made it easier for them to then add other symptom management strategies.

Here is a closer look at a few key nutrients for PMS:

Vitamin B-6
Also known as pyridoxine, vitamin B-6 helps metabolize proteins and hormones and helps regulate the central nervous system. It also appears to be important in the regulation of mood swings, irritability, fatigue, and fluid retention. Studies on its use for PMS, however, have produced mixed results. The recommended daily intake for vitamin B-6 is 1.3 mg. per day for premenopausal women between the ages of 19 and 50 but keep in mind that this level is set with the goal of avoiding deficiencies in the general population, not for managing symptoms and enhancing health. If you do supplement your diet, be sure you don't exceed 200 mg. of vitamin B-6 daily; otherwise, taking large amounts over an extended period of time could result in neurological side effects such as numbness or tingling in the extremities. Good food sources include: soy-based meat substitutes such as veggie burgers, meats, fish, poultry, grains and cereals (especially the fortified ones), sweet potatoes, bananas, and avocados.

Vitamin E
While there's little scientific evidence that vitamin E will reduce the pain that's associated with cystic changes in the breasts, some health-

care practitioners recommend this measure to their patients and report that it helps. If you decide to try this approach, the recommendation for breast tenderness is 400 IU of vitamin E daily; don't exceed 1,000 IU per day. Good food sources include wheat germ, whole grains, seeds and nuts, broccoli, turnip greens, and vegetable oils.

Magnesium

Not only does magnesium promote proper heart function and energy production, but it is also calming to the nervous system. And it has been found to relieve muscle spasms, constipation, and symptoms of PMS. In fact, there's been some suggestion that women with PMS have lowered levels of magnesium in their blood cells, despite having normal levels outside those cells. The recommended daily intake for magnesium is 310 mg. for women ages 19 to 30 and 320 mg. for women over 30. Good food sources include beet greens, Swiss chard, lima beans, black beans, tofu, pineapple, raspberries, almonds, sunflower seeds, rye flour, and fortified whole-grain cereals and breads.

Potassium

It's one of the primary minerals inside the body's cells, and research has linked low levels of potassium with fatigue and low energy. After all, potassium is required to convert glucose to glycogen, a stored form of energy; it also produces an electrical charge that stimulates the muscles to work properly and, along with phosphorus, sends oxygen to the brain to maintain alertness and cognitive functioning. Good food sources include: apricots, beet greens, lima beans, Swiss chard, winter squash, cantaloupe, orange juice, black beans, lentils, dried fruits, cherries, grapes, bananas, potatoes, and milk.

Calcium

Aside from its claim to fame as a bone-building nutrient, calcium is a calming agent that is depleted by stress. In a randomized controlled trial, women with PMS experienced a 50 percent reduction in their symptoms while taking 1,200 mg. of calcium daily; moreover, food cravings and pain decreased by 54 percent. The theory is that calcium supplementation may act by repairing an underlying deficit, suppressing parathyroid hormone secretion, and ultimately reducing neuromuscular irritability and vascular reactivity. The current daily recommendation for premenopausal women is 1,000 mg.; don't exceed 2,500 mg., or you could experience constipation, muscle spasms, or an increased risk of kidney stones. Good food sources include: dairy products, canned salmon and sardines, tofu, broccoli, and fortified orange juice.

Rather than trying to get more of these into your diet by taking specific nutrient supplements, it's better to take a multivitamin and mineral supplement (with the exception of calcium). Otherwise, it's a bit like playing supplement roulette because you'll be gambling on getting the right amounts of the right nutrients—but not too much. Also, because these nutrients operate together in the body, it's likely that they have a synergistic beneficial effect on symptoms. That's why it's smart to take a multivitamin and mineral supplement that offers a wide array of nutrients in their fully recommended amounts.

What should you look for in a well-rounded supplement? For starters, choose a multivitamin and mineral supplement that provides about 100 percent but no more of the recommended intakes for most nutrients. You'll find the percentages listed on the label. Whether you go the generic or the name brand route is up to you; generally, both are equally safe and effective. But do look for the USP designation, which means that the formula meets the standards set by the United States Pharmocopeia for quality and purity. Take this vitamin-mineral supplement once a day—preferably with food since some of the fat-soluble vitamins are better absorbed with a meal that contains some fat—beginning on the first day of your period. Don't use this supplement as license to indulge in poor eating habits, though: As their name suggests, these formulas are designed to be supplements to—rather than replacements for—a healthy diet.

Since you can't get all the calcium you need from a multivitamin and mineral supplement—calcium is simply too bulky of a nutrient to fit into the tablet without making it into a horse pill—you may want to take a separate calcium supplement. If you're getting two or more servings of dairy foods daily, plus another serving of a calcium-rich food such as calcium-enriched orange juice, you may not need to take a supplement. If your calcium intake isn't what it should be from food sources, it's best to take no more than 500 to 600 mg. in supplements at a time because the body has a hard time absorbing more than this amount. Whether you choose calcium carbonate or calcium citrate is up to you. A recent study from Creighton University in Omaha, Nebraska, found that both forms are equally well absorbed. (Calcium carbonate is best absorbed with food, however.) Choose whichever form agrees with you—and take one of the tablets at night.

As far as PMS supplements go, in recent years, several PMS formulas have begun appearing on drugstore and health-food-store shelves. Most of these are high in vitamin B-6 as well as magnesium and calcium but offer other nutrients as well, and most of these formulas suggest that you take up to eight tablets per day. In trying to determine the effectiveness of these supplements, I selected two of the most common PMS formulas on the market in the early 1990s—Ultravite, a generic version of Optivite, a multivitamin-mineral supplement developed by Guy Abraham, M.D., as a nutritional treatment for PMS; and the Schiff PMS 1 Nutritional Supplement—for research purposes. I selected these formulas because they had safe dosages of vitamin B-6, required taking the fewest number of pills per day, had approximately the same formulas, and were widely available. In a clinical trial I conducted, half of the women started on the Schiff formula and half started on the Ultravite; more women changed from Ultravite to the Schiff because of the smaller size of the pills or because the Ultravite disagreed with them.

Because the Schiff PMS 1 Nutritional Supplement is well-tolerated by most women and requires taking no more than eight small gelatin capsules, that's the one I recommend most often. Whether you choose this brand or another, what you want to look for in any PMS formula is one that contains vitamin B-6 along with the entire complex of B vitamins, magnesium, and calcium, at the very least. Ideally, you'd want the formula to look something like this*:

---

* Note: Some of these amounts exceed the upper limits recommended by the National Academy of Sciences if you take the maximum dosage of the Schiff PMS 1 Formula—meaning, all eight capsules in a day. Some of the women in my research started with four capsules a day, which would yield half of these amounts; as time went on, more than half of the women winded up taking four to six capsules a day during the premenstrual phase. If you do ingest the maximum dosage—eight capsules per day—for half of your menstrual cycle, the higher amounts aren't likely to pose a health risk since you won't be doing this all the time.

Vitamin A . . . . .15,000 I.U.

Vitamin D . . . . .100 I.U.

Vitamin E . . . . .600 I.U.

Vitamin C . . . . .1,000 mg

Folic acid . . . . .200 mcg

Thiamine (Vitamin B-1) . . . . .50 mg

Riboflavin (Vitamin B-2) . . . . . . .50 mg

Niacin .50 mg

Vitamin B-6 . . . . .200 mg

Vitamin B-12 . . . . .50 mcg

Biotin .30 mcg

Pantothenic acid . . . . .50 mg

Calcium . . . . .150 mg

Magnesium . . . . .300 mg

Iodine .150 mcg

Iron . . . . .15 mg

Zinc . . . . .25 mg

Manganese . . . . .10 mg

Potassium . . . . .100 mg

Selenium . . . . .25 mcg

Chromium . . . . .100 mcg

Here's how the whole vitamin protocol works: On day 14 or about midway through your menstrual cycle, you should stop taking your regular multivitamin and start taking the PMS formula. Divide up the recommended number of daily tablets and start by taking one-third of the tablets at breakfast and one-third of them at lunchtime. If symptoms don't seem to be improving and if you haven't experienced side effects with this dose, you could take the final one-third of the recommended tablets at dinner or in the mid-afternoon if you notice sleep problems at night. Always take the supplements with food because you're more likely to experience stomach upset if you take them on an empty stomach. If you smoke, try to refrain for at least an hour after taking any nutritional supplement because nicotine decreases the transit time of food in the bowel and decreases absorption of the nutrients. Whatever you do, do not exceed the maximum number of pills per day. If you continue to have PMS symptoms a few days into your period, it's fine to continue taking the PMS formula for a few more days. Just be sure to switch back to the regular multivitamin with mineral and stop taking the PMS formula by the end of your period.

In addition to the vitamin and mineral regimen, it's wise to include more foods that are friends to PMS and to get rid of the foes. Here's what you'll want to aim for:

Increase your consumption of complex carbs:

Carbohydrates are the body's main source of energy. With the exception of fiber, all carbohydrates are transformed into blood sugar (primarily glucose), which triggers the release of insulin. Aided by other nutrients, insulin allows blood sugar to enter the cells of the body, where it supplies energy to the muscles and other tissues. There are two types of carbohydrates—simple forms (which are sugars such as glucose, fructose, lactose, and sucrose) and complex carbs (which are primarily starches). Generally, complex carbohydrates are digested more slowly and make you feel full for longer than simple carbohydrates do. They also produce a more modest spike in blood sugar, and this slow, steady rise in blood sugar may help keep your energy and mood on a more even keel.

Time after time, studies have found that women with PMS crave carbohydrates—and it's probably for good reason: A desire to spark biochemical changes that will have a calming effect on the brain and body. After all, some researchers believe that eating carbohydrates seems to set in motion a cascade of events that lead to an increase in serotonin levels in the brain, which can produce feelings of emotional stability and tranquility. In research scientist Judith Wurtman's study, for example, after the women with PMS ate a carbohydrate-rich meal in the evening, they experienced a drop in feelings of depression, tension, anger, confusion, sadness, and fatigue and an increase in alertness and calmness. Since synthesis of serotonin in the brain increases after a high carbohydrate intake, Wurtman's theory is that women with premenstrual syndrome may overeat carbohydrates in an attempt to improve their downbeat moods by raising serotonin levels. Similarly, in a study at Massachusetts General Hospital in Boston, women with PMS who increased their intake of complex carbohydrates—in this case, by consuming a carbohydrate-rich beverage—experienced a significant decrease in premenstrual symptoms such as depression, anger, confusion, and food cravings.

While complex carbohydrates should be the mainstay of any healthy diet, women with PMS may want to increase their intake to 60 to 70 percent of their day's calories. How to get more complex carbs? While white bread and white rice are considered complex carbohydrates, the whole-grain variety of complex carbohydrates is healthier. Look for items whose labels claim they contain 100 percent whole wheat or whole grains. Don't be fooled by foods that are labeled as "wheat"; these are often made with refined flour that has the bran processed out of it. The unrefined whole-wheat flour that is used to make whole-wheat bread, by contrast, still has the high-fiber, nutrient-dense bran intact, and it's rich in vitamins, minerals, and phytochemicals (disease-fighting substances that occur naturally in plants). Think in terms of brown foods over white foods—brown rice instead of white rice, whole-wheat pasta instead of semolina, and so on—and you'll be headed in the right direction.

Within the complex carbohydrate family, you also may want to choose foods that have a lower glycemic index (GI)—it reflects the effect of various carbohydrate foods on blood sugar—whenever possible, during the premenstrual phase. Carbohydrates are considered to have a high GI if they are quickly broken down during digestion and lead to a rapid spike in blood sugar. Carbohydrates that have a low GI, on the other hand, are broken down slowly and gradually release glucose into the bloodstream. Using the GI to guide food choices during the latter half of your menstrual cycle may help you avoid wide fluctuations in blood sugar levels and, hence, energy and mood. Here are some examples of how you might make low GI choices in terms of complex carbohydrates:

Choose a 100 percent bran cereal or oatmeal instead of corn flakes.

Choose pumpernickel or rye bread over white or wheat bread.

Choose fruits such as apples, pears, and plums over tropical fruits like bananas, mangoes, papaya, and watermelon.

Choose beans and legumes over starchy vegetables like corn and potatoes.

Whether or not you choose to follow the glycemic index, do incorporate more complex carbohydrates into all your meals. For breakfast, try switching to whole-grain or multi-grain bagels or bread, English muffins, or hot cereal; or try unsweetened whole-grain cold cereals such as shredded wheat or 100 percent bran flakes. For lunch, items such as lentil, split pea, black bean, or navy bean soups, bean-filled burritos, or a baked potato with low-fat yogurt and a sprinkling of parmesan cheese provide a healthy mix of complex carbohydrates and protein. And for dinner, whole-grain pastas, brown rice, cracked wheat such as tabbouleh, or tortillas can provide the basis for a complex-carbohydrate-rich meal. Between-meal snacks might include low-fat microwave popcorn, brown-rice cakes, whole-grain crackers, fresh fruits, dried fruits and nuts, or vegetables with a yogurt or bean dip.

Limit simple sugars:

When PMS strikes, you may feel like getting cozy with a box of cookies or a pint of fudge brownie ice cream, but it's a bad idea. Whether they come in the form of candy bars, sodas, donuts, or sugary cereals, simple sugars act as stimulants that can increase premenstrual symptoms and cause the body to release additional insulin from the pancreas, which can precipitate a rebound of low blood sugar and produce symptoms such as fatigue and irritability. The body, and especially the brain, needs a consistent source of glucose to function smoothly so it's primed to swing into action to regulate the highs and lows of blood sugar. Because refined carbohydrates and simple sugars get dumped into the blood-stream very quickly, this rapid spike in blood sugar triggers the secretion of insulin. Not only can excessively high levels of insulin trigger the body to store calories as fat, which can increase the risk of heart disease and diabetes, but they can also stimulate appetite and sugar cravings, in particular. When you must consume simple sugars, do so with a regular meal or with some protein to help stabilize your blood sugar.

Of course, sometimes it's just too difficult to resist the lure of the pantry or vending machine during the premenstrual phase. You may be wondering whether it's possible to have whatever it is that you crave without losing control and worsening your symptoms. The good news is, it is. Here are several strategies to help you indulge while still exercising dietary damage control:

- If you have a yen for chocolate, chips, or candy, your best bet is to eat one or two small bites very slowly. Chew methodically and savor the taste. Don't do anything else except enjoy the taste and texture of what you're eating.

- If you can't seem to limit yourself to just one or two bites, then cut up the item into bite-size pieces and wrap them up and freeze them for future premenstrual cravings.

- If your craving is for something sweet, such as cookies or ice cream, you could suck on hard candy, have a mug of hot chocolate or herb tea with honey, dust a rice cake with cocoa powder, or dip apple wedges into two tablespoons' worth of fat-free chocolate or butterscotch sauce, instead. If these measures don't do the trick, have a small amount of what you truly crave along with a little protein and drink a glass of water afterwards to balance the sugar. If your cravings are for salty items, drink two glasses of water after indulging to reduce water retention.

What to do if you overindulge:

- Drink two to four glasses of water and/or herbal tea to help flush out the salt and prevent water retention.

- Think about what caused you to overeat so that you'll be alert to such triggers in the future.

- Don't beat yourself up about this slip. Forgive yourself and move forward.

Restrict your salt intake:
Research has found that a high salt intake can produce temporary weight gain and bloating, especially during the premenstrual phase, because of the increased levels of progesterone and anti-diuretic hormone that are associated with the luteal phase of the menstrual cycle. Plus, a heightened response to stress can increase fluid retention due to activation of the adrenal glands. Some women appear to be more sensitive to the effects of sodium than others. If you're prone to fluid retention, reducing your salt intake while increasing your water intake is the safest, most effective way of avoiding the bloating blues. The average American diet contains up to 6,900 mg. of sodium per day, the amount contained in about three teaspoons of salt. Your best bet is to aim for no more than 2,400 mg. during the premenstrual phase of your cycle, or, if you suffer from considerable fluid retention premenstrually,

try to limit your salt intake to between 500 and 2,000 mg. per day from ovulation until your period begins.

It's not as simple as letting go of the salt shaker, though. High levels of sodium are hidden in all sorts of foods including processed items such as canned vegetables or frozen entrees, luncheon meats, smoked or pickled fish, snack foods like potato or tortilla chips, and salad dressings. To avoid such salt-laden traps, use fresh vegetables and salt-free seasoning, whenever possible, and buy unsalted crackers or low-salt microwave popcorn for snacks.

Include some protein in every meal:

Protein is important in the PMS picture for several reasons. Protein-rich foods can help buffer blood sugar swings because protein takes longer to digest and, hence, provides a more gradual rise in blood sugar. In addition, the body needs a regular supply of protein for the production of glucagon, which is responsible for releasing sugar, fat, and protein from the cells for use as fuel and as the building blocks in the brain that serve as precursors to the production of neurotransmitters such as serotonin. But only moderate amounts of dietary protein are needed for these purposes—and incorporating protein in each meal is actually quite simple: For breakfast, you might have toast with peanut butter or hot cereal made with milk instead of water; for lunch, you could have chili with beans or whole-wheat pita bread with hummus; and for dinner, you could make soft-shelled tacos with ground turkey or Spanish rice with beans.

This is an instance where more is not necessarily better, though: Too much protein can leach calcium and other minerals from the bone or interfere with mineral absorption. Moreover, research has suggested that high amounts of protein—more than 85 grams per day, which is the equivalent of a 12-ounce T-bone steak—can increase the risk of kidney problems. So it's best to stay in the moderate range.

Eat smaller, more frequent meals:

Rather than sticking with three square meals per day, try having smaller, carbohydrate-based mini-meals up to six times per day to ensure a smooth flow of nutrients to the body's cells and to avoid dramatic fluctuations in blood sugar levels. When you go for long periods without eating, this can stimulate the adrenal system to release stress hormones such as adrenaline and cortisol—since the body perceives this scarcity of food as a physical threat—and lead to low blood-glucose levels. As a result, you may experience an increase in symptoms such as fatigue, jitteriness, weakness, or headaches, especially during the premenstrual period when blood-sugar levels already have more ups and downs.

That's why it's a good idea for women with PMS to eat something—whether it's a snack or a mini-meal—every two to three hours all month long. Following this schedule can help you avoid blood-sugar swings—not to mention the fatigue, shakiness, cravings, and other accompanying symptoms—and maintain a higher, more consistent level of energy. In fact, a study at Dr. Katharina Dalton's PMS clinic in London found that consuming a small portion of a starchy carbohydrate six times per day helped to relieve the severity of PMS in 70 percent of women.

How to squeeze in all this food? It's easier than you might think. You can either divide the day's meals into five or six mini-meals or simply include a mid-morning and a mid-afternoon snack to your usual routine and downsize your portion sizes at breakfast, lunch, and dinner. Either way, it's important to have nutritious snacks such as baby carrots with a low-fat yogurt dip or hummus, soy nuts or trail mix, or string cheese and rice cakes available at troublesome times—while cooking dinner for the family or commuting home after a long day at work, for example. Just be sure that you don't go longer than three hours without eating.

Energy-Boosting Elixirs

If you don't eat breakfast but want an easy energy drink or you want a late-afternoon pick-me-up, my own concoction, **The Green Drink**, is a good option that will help you get down your vitamins. Here's how to make it: In a blender, combine one cup of pineapple chunks or juice, a large handful of raw spinach, a banana, ½ cup plain yogurt, and some papaya chunks if you have problems with your digestion. Add two tablespoons of soy powder, wheat germ, or rice bran, and blend until thick and frothy. Pour into a tall glass and serve.

If you feel as though fatigue is dragging you down, try a **potassium-rich smoothie** for breakfast or a mid-afternoon energy boost. In a blender, combine ½ cup skim milk, 1 cup low-fat vanilla yogurt, ¾ cup fresh or frozen blackberries or strawberries, 1 banana, and 1 tablespoon honey (optional). Blend until thick and frothy—add a handful of ice for extra froth—then serve. With either beverage, drink a toast to your health!

Drink more water:

It's the most abundant substance in the body, accounting for 50 to 75 percent of your body weight, yet many women don't give water the respect it deserves. Not only is this indispensable nutrient vital to cellular processes throughout the body, but good old H_2O also aids digestion, assists with the absorption and transportation of nutrients, helps maintain the body's temperature and electrolyte balance, and keeps your skin and other membranes moist, among other functions. Of course, water is also necessary for the metabolism and excretion of bodily waste. In order for the kidneys to excrete water, they must add salt (or sodium) to it, so drinking water leads to the elimination of water and salt.

While there is no official minimum daily requirement for water, most nutritionists recommend drinking at least eight 8-ounce glasses of water per day. If the taste of plain water doesn't appeal to you, consider increasing your water intake by adding lemon or orange slices to your H_2O and consuming plenty of decaffeinated or herbal teas and watered-down fruit juices. During the premenstrual phase of your cycle, you may want to increase your water consumption to eight 12-ounce glasses (or 96 ounces). It may seem counterintuitive but the more water you drink, the more salt and waste you will excrete and the less bloating and swelling you will have.

Eliminate—or at least limit—your caffeine intake:

Over the years, caffeine has been blamed as a contributing culprit to numerous health problems from heart disease to cancer, from miscarriages to breast lumps and birth defects. While moderate caffeine consumption—defined as 300 mg., or two to three 8-ounce cups of regular coffee per day—has been exonerated from blame for these problems, caffeine can exacerbate PMS symptoms. Large amounts can even induce anxiety in healthy individuals. This doesn't mean that you have to deprive yourself of your cherished cappuccino or chocolate, altogether. But you should limit your consumption of caffeine-containing foods and beverages during the premenstrual phase of your cycle.

Rather than severely curtailing your caffeine intake, which could cause symptoms of withdrawal, start by gradually decreasing your daily intake of caffeine—perhaps by having half-caffeinated and half-decaffeinated coffee or by substituting decaffeinated tea or colas for your favorite versions of these. Although chocolate contains much less caffeine than either coffee or tea, solid, dark chocolate can contain as much caffeine as half a cup of brewed coffee or black tea. A quick look at the caffeine content of various foods and beverages: 5 ounces of regular drip coffee contains 60 to 180 mg.; 5 ounces of tea contains 20 to 50 mg.; 12 ounces of cola has up to 50 mg.; 8 ounces of chocolate milk has about 5 mg.; 1 ounce of dark chocolate has up to 35 mg. whereas 1 ounce of milk chocolate has up to 15 mg.

Sharply curtail your consumption of alcohol:
When you're feeling all revved up with nowhere to go during the premenstrual phase, it may be tempting to turn to a glass of wine or two with the hope that alcohol will calm you down. It won't. The reality is, alcohol can actually worsen physical and emotional symptoms of PMS.

As Tanya, 35, a chef, confesses: "I used to drink four or five glasses of wine before my period to help me calm down but then I would say things I didn't mean. While charting my symptoms, I realized that I would crave alcohol for a few days right before my period. I tried eating more frequently, eating more whole grains, and drinking a lot of water—and that helped reduce my cravings."

Complicating the matter, women appear to be more susceptible to the effects of alcohol premenstrually than at other times of the month: Research has found that when women are given an equal amount of alcohol in both premenstrual and postmenstrual weeks, they show an impaired tolerance for alcohol—meaning, their blood alcohol level is higher and they register the effects sooner—during the premenstrual week. Your best bet is to limit or eliminate alcohol during the premenstrual days. If you enjoy unwinding after a stressful day with a glass of wine or a beer, choose non-alcoholic versions in the week before your period—or have a wine spritzer, with half the usual quantity of wine mixed with seltzer.

Eat more amino acids:
Increasing your intake of foods that are high in amino acids such as tyrosine and tryptophan can help relieve premenstrual symptoms such as fatigue, irritability, and depression. Tyrosine can help improve concentration and suppress an overactive appetite. A precursor to energizing biochemicals such as adrenaline and dopamine, tyrosine-rich foods can pave the way for increased energy and feelings of well-being. Tryp-

tophan, by contrast, forms the building blocks for the feel-good brain chemical serotonin, which can improve mood and induce feelings of calmness.

Good sources of tyrosine include cheddar cheese, low-fat cottage cheese, almonds, pumpkin and sesame seeds, chicken and roasted turkey, plain low-fat yogurt, soy milk, beans, and peas. Foods that are rich in tryptophan include canned tuna or canned salmon, ham, various cuts of beef, turkey, low-fat cottage cheese, skim milk, and lima beans. As far as PMS goes, research hasn't pinpointed an ideal amount of either amino acid but you can't go wrong aiming for 750 mg. of tyrosine and 1,000 mg. of tryptophan per day. This is easily achieved by consuming half a cup of cottage cheese or 3½ ounces of roasted turkey (the dark meat) or 1 cup of split pea soup and a cup of low-fat fruit-flavored yogurt, in the case of tyrosine. To get ample amounts of tryptophan from your diet, you could eat 1 cup of low-fat cottage cheese plus 3½ ounces of canned salmon and 5 ounces of roasted turkey breast over the course of a day. (Some women try to increase their intake of these amino acids and others by taking supplements. For more information about these options, see Chapter Eleven.)

MORE FOOD FOR THOUGHT

Remember: Changing your dietary habits can be difficult, especially if your current eating style has become ingrained over the course of years or decades. And if you don't have the support of family members or friends—who may find these changes threatening, in some way—it can be that much more challenging to make these shifts. Try to determine the approach—whether it's an overhaul of your diet or gradual changes—that makes the most sense for you. Be realistic about what you can really do so that you'll be setting yourself up for success. It may help to get in touch with your true eating habits before trying to embark on these changes. To do that, you may want to keep a food diary for a few days, during the week and over the weekend, before and after your period. (You'll find a sample form in the Appendix.)

If it's easier, don't be afraid to make small, incremental changes to your eating habits. Even these count as changes, and they could make a difference in how you feel. At first, many women in my PMS studies made dietary changes only during the premenstrual phases of their menstrual cycles because this made them feel less deprived than instituting these changes all month long would have. After feeling the effects of upgrading their eating habits, though, most of the women integrated these changes into their month-long and now life-long dietary practices. Keep in mind, though, that it may take two to four months for you to see results from dietary changes. Look at cookbooks or cooking magazines to get new ideas about how to prepare these PMS-friendly foods. By tinkering with your diet and expanding your culinary repertoire, you're likely to find a palatable way to curb your premenstrual symptoms.

YOUR ASSIGNMENT:

Spend a little time thinking about what goals you'd like to set for modifying your diet. This will help you make feasible choices and anticipate what might be involved. To get the ideas flowing, answer the following questions:

☐ What specific changes are you willing to make in your eating pattern?

☐ Have you tried to make similar dietary changes in the past? If so, what were the results and how did you feel while trying to make those changes?

☐ Think about your typical eating patterns as well as when and where you're most vulnerable to overeating in response to cravings. Then consider what you could do, instead, to counteract those cravings.

☐ List as many concrete actions and ideas as you can for meeting your dietary goals.

☐ Now think about potential obstacles that might stand in your way (time constraints, unsupportive people, negative self-talk, and the like)—and how you'll deal with them.

☐ Who will you ask to help or support you in achieving your goals?

5

Exercising Your Options

When a woman is feeling like something the cat dragged in, courtesy of PMS, she'd probably rather lie on the couch with a pint of rocky road ice cream or a jumbo-size bag of potato chips than head to the gym. But you should think twice about this choice. Why? Because regular aerobic exercise can ease many premenstrual symptoms as well as helping you feel like you can cope better. After all, regular aerobic exercise is a central ingredient of good physical and emotional health. It tones the muscles, strengthens the bones, improves the function of your heart and lungs, helps prevent constipation, reduces the level of stress-related hormones that are circulating through your body, and promotes a renewed sense of well-being and vitality.

Moreover, research suggests that the benefits of a regular exercise program may directly alleviate some premenstrual symptoms such as bloating, abdominal and muscle cramps, headaches, and lower back pain. Moderate physical activity has also been found to improve sleep, reduce fatigue, and improve cognitive abilities. How can exercise work such magic in so many different ways? Physical activity, as you undoubtedly know, increases your heart rate and blood flow, which means that more oxygen and nutrients are supplied to the lungs, the heart, and the muscles, especially the large muscle groups. In addition, regular, moderate exercise can enhance immune function. And when you sweat, you will help the body rid itself of fluid retention and toxins. Moreover, many studies have shown that levels of endorphins—the body's natural opiates—rise in the bloodstream and the brain during vigorous exercise, creating an enhanced sense of well-being.

Exercise also may indirectly ease emotional symptoms such as anxiety and irritability by boosting your self-esteem as well as your ability to cope with everyday hassles and major catastrophes. In fact, a recent study from Duke University Medical Center in Durham, North Carolina, compared the effects of exercise treatment with antidepressants or a combination of the two among 156 people with major depressive disorder; after ten months, those who continued working out regularly had lower relapse rates than did those who'd been taking antidepressants. Moreover, research has found that women who exercise regularly report feelings of well-being, improved mood, fewer memory and concentration problems, reduced anxiety, and improved perceptions of overall well-being and quality of life. Intuitively, all of this makes sense if you think about it: After all, when you feel physically fit and strong, you are likely to feel better able to emotionally handle whatever stresses and strains come your way. Another benefit of exercise is that it's a time-out or distraction from the hassles of daily living, a chance to get away for 30 minutes or more and clear your mind. All of these findings are encouraging, particularly because research suggests that it is not necessary to reach peak physical fitness for the stress-reducing, mood-lifting benefits of exercise to kick in.

Most studies that have examined the effects of exercise on PMS have investigated aerobic exercise as a treatment. In one study, previously sedentary women embarked on a six-month running program; by the end of the training program, they experienced significantly fewer premenstrual symptoms, including decreased fluid retention, breast discomfort, and premenstrual depression and anxiety.

In my own research, two-thirds of the women found aerobic exercise to be very helpful in easing premenstrual symptoms and one-third found yoga to be especially beneficial for PMS relief. By the long-term follow-up—18 to 24 months after launching their programs—35 percent of the women were doing aerobic exercise on a daily basis and 50 percent of the women were doing a combination of yoga and aerobic exercise each day. The primary types of exercise women used were walking, jogging, aerobic dance, and swimming. Many of the women had a hard time getting started if they did not already exercise on a regular basis. They knew that exercise would help them feel better both physically and emotionally; they just found it difficult to fit regular workouts into their busy lives. For them, exercise was either just one more thing to do during a hectic day; or, because they felt bad physically and emotionally, they just couldn't get themselves going when their PMS was at its most severe.

For women suffering from PMS, participating in physical activity throughout the month but modifying the regimen one to two weeks before the arrival of their periods may work best to alleviate symptoms. Combining regular aerobic exercise with relaxation or meditative strategies, especially during the premenstrual phase, may actually multiply the effects on mood and well-being. Many women in my research substituted yoga or stretching for more vigorous activities during the premenstrual or menstrual weeks. Or, if you love vigorous aerobic exercise but still want to relax, you can take ten minutes to float on your back after swimming or to stroll along a favorite path after running. One way or another, the vast majority of the women in my research found that continuing to move, even when their PMS was flaring up, was beneficial for their physical and emotional well-being. As one woman notes, "When I am exercising regularly, I notice that my mood is more stable all month long and my menstrual cramps aren't so severe."

THE RIGHT EXERCISE FORMULA

Exercise doesn't have to be jarring or intense if it is to help PMS. Of course, it can be aerobic—meaning it activates your cardiovascular and respiratory systems—in the form of running, biking, or skiing, for example, but kinder, gentler forms of exercise such as stretching, or performing yoga or Pilates can also create feelings of calm and ease premenstrual symptoms. Moreover, a combination of mind-body activities in the form of gardening, weight-training, or going for a leisurely walk also count in the PMS-easing equation. This approach to exercise is also supported by recent research on the prevention of chronic diseases and the promotion of health and well-being: Rather than emphasizing intense physical exercise, the focus is on incorporating more movement into all aspects of your life—work, play, home, or school.

Most of the exercise recommendations have focused on cardiovascular fitness, which, until recently, meant increasing your heart rate for 30 to 45 minutes at a stretch, three to four times a week. Not only does this seem like an overwhelming goal for many busy women—or like a Herculean task when you are experiencing pain, discomfort, or a case of the doldrums premenstrually—but the latest research suggests that more moderate exercise can have very positive effects. The ongoing Nurses Health Study, for example, found that women who walk briskly for three hours a week are equally well protected from heart disease as women who engage in more vigorous activities. Other research has found that regular, moderate exercise—in the form of walking, in particular—is associated with improved immune function and fewer upper respiratory infections.

To be considered aerobic, an activity must use large muscle groups and be intense enough to condition the heart and lungs. Whether you choose to walk briskly, run, bike, swim, row, climb stairs, or ski, your body will naturally increase its consumption of oxygen during these activities and challenge your heart and lungs to work harder. That's why aerobic exercise is often called cardiorespiratory conditioning. During this sort of activity, your heart rate should get into its target zone— between 60 and 80 percent of your maximum heart rate—for at least 20 to 30 minutes. (There is little added benefit to exercising beyond this 80 percent capacity—and it could be dangerous, in some people.)

■ *Your Heart Rate's Target Zone* ■

To calculate your target zone, start by subtracting your age from 220—this number estimates your maximum heart rate in beats per minute. Now, multiply the resulting number by .60 to gauge the lower limit of your target zone and multiply your maximum heart rate by .80 to figure out the upper limit. Here's how the formula would work for a 34-year-old woman:

220–34 (age) = 186 (Maximum HR in beats per minute)

186 × .60 = 111.6 (lower limit of target zone)

186 × .80 = 148.8 (upper limit of target zone)

Her target heart-rate zone: 112 to 149 beats per minute (rounded off)

If you stay within this window, you'll be exercising at the ideal aerobic intensity. You can determine if you're in this zone by taking a break while exercising and immediately checking your pulse on your wrist: Count the number of beats in 15 seconds then multiply this number by four to gauge your heart rate in beats per minute. If your heart rate exceeds the upper limit of your target zone, reduce the intensity or pace of what you're doing. If it's below the lower limit, step up the pace or intensity if you want to reap weight-loss or cardiovascular benefits from your workout.

How you structure your exercise program is up to you, and it will depend largely on your goals. If you want to improve your endurance, for example, you might choose to do vigorous activities—such as running, kayaking, long-distance walking, or biking at a fast pace—more frequently (meaning at least four times per week) for 30 to 60 minutes. If you want to get in the habit of engaging in regular, moderate exercise, you might aim to walk, bike, skate, hike, or play tennis at a moderate pace for at least 30 minutes on most days of the week. If you want to enhance your flexibility, you'll want to select activities such as yoga, tai chi, chi gong, or stretching routines that move your joints and muscles through their full range of motion and perform them anywhere from four to seven times per week.

On the other hand, if you want to lose weight, you'd want to exercise at least five days per week, according to recommendations from the American College of Sports Medicine. And if you want to build or maintain muscle mass and endurance, you should choose strength-training activities—weight-lifting, resistance training with exercise bands, or moving your body against gravity by doing push-ups and the like—and perform these two to three times per week. Not only does strength training help tone your muscles, rather than making them bulky, but it also confers a weight-management benefit. Lean muscle burns calories at a faster rate than body fat does: A pound of muscle burns 35 to 50 calories per day compared to only two calories per day for body fat. So when you gain lean muscle through strength-training activities, you'll also gain a metabolic boost, which can help you lose weight, if that's your goal.

As far as PMS goes, the aim is to get enough exercise at the right intensity but not to overdo it. When you exercise strenuously on a consistent basis, you might lose weight and body fat; you could fall into a state of energy imbalance (if your calorie intake doesn't compensate for the calories you burn through exercise); or you could alter the production of hormones in your body—any of which can cause disturbances to your menstrual cycle. Another hidden hazard: Over-training can lead to mood disturbances because of its stress-inducing mechanism, which could potentially exacerbate premenstrual symptoms. Your best bet is to follow the course of moderation.

Fortunately, you can combine aerobic exercise and flexibility training in the same workout—by performing gentle stretches before and after walking, for example. In fact, to prevent injuries, it's always smart to begin an exercise session with a five to ten-minute warm-up period to increase blood flow and allow the muscles to warm up before moving into the aerobic part of the session and to end with a cool-down period, followed by five to ten minutes of stretching. This will allow your heart rate, blood pressure, and body temperature a chance to gradually return to normal. The cool-down period is also a prime opportunity for enhancing flexibility through stretching since your muscles are warm and limber by then. Be sure to drink plenty of water before, during, and after a workout to ensure adequate hydration and recovery from exercise.

WHAT'S STOPPING YOU?

It's a truism that applies to most things in life—and exercise is no exception: If you expect to fail, you probably will because, consciously or not, you'll set up psychological barriers that will prevent you from succeeding. Self-critical or negative thoughts can actually have effects on neurotransmitters in the brain that can work against you. If you think you are too tired to exercise, for example, there's a good chance you will wind up feeling too tired to get moving. Instead of setting up that self-fulfilling prophecy, you can reinforce positive beliefs about exercise—that it can make you feel more alert or reduce the severity of your premenstrual symptoms, for example.

Debbie, 35, a human resources manager, had never had a good experience with exercise and even though she knew it would be good for her, she had put off adding exercise to her personal PMS program for months. To get over her mental block, she started visualizing an activity she enjoyed—hiking along the beach with a close friend—every day for a week. The reverie proved to be so pleasant that Debbie decided to actually go hiking the following week. She loved it and began making a point of going for a long hike every weekend. Later, she added 20 minutes of yoga each night during the week. As she went through the moves, she focused on how good she felt while doing them. Within a few weeks, she began to feel comfortable with the idea of trying other forms of exercise. "I used to think of exercise as a chore," she explains. "But once I found activities I actually enjoy, it became something I looked forward to."

If you want to set yourself up for success, here's Rule Number One: Have realistic expectations. The truth is, you may not feel the benefits of exercise right away. On the contrary, exercise may feel more like a chore than a panacea at first. That's to be expected if you've been relatively inactive until now. In fact, if you've been sedentary, it may take a little while for exercise to feel even remotely comfortable and enjoyable. (Keep in mind: If you have underlying health problems or risk factors for heart disease, it's a good idea to consult your health-care provider before beginning any exercise program.)

To avoid trying to tackle too much too soon, ease into your exercise regimen by starting at a comfortable pace and increasing the intensity and duration of your workouts as you feel ready. Build up your workouts gradually, increasing the length or intensity of your workouts by no more than 10 percent per week. Over-training can make you feel exhausted, sick, tired, or achy. If you feel this way after working out, reduce the length or intensity of what you're doing until you can come away from it feeling refreshed. If that doesn't work, consider switching to a milder, gentler form of exercise that you can perform for a longer period of time without stressing your adrenal glands and the rest of your body.

When it comes to making exercise a habit, half the battle is to find activities that you enjoy, ones that don't feel like another chore on an already overburdened "To Do" list. The only way to do this is through trial and error—by trying various physical activities in different venues and seeing what suits your personal style and comfort level. Another large part of the battle is to find the time to actually carry out your good intentions. To that end, you'll need the support of your spouse and family. You'll also need to choose a time of day that makes sense for you—even if it's only 15 minutes, to start—and to treat your scheduled workout as if it were just as crucial as an important business or hair appointment.

Even if you're tired, remind yourself that being active will give you more energy. Then, bargain with yourself—or bribe yourself, if need be—to exercise. Elizabeth, 36, a writer who confesses to often feeling like a slug when she's premenstrual, uses what she calls "the ten-minute rule" to get herself moving. "When I really don't feel like going for a run, I force myself to do it for at least ten minutes," she explains. "I remind myself that I can stand just about anything for ten minutes so there's no reason not to go. The rule is that if it feels terrible after ten minutes, I have permission to quit. But I hardly ever do. Once I've been running for ten minutes, I usually feel more invigorated and want to keep going." (If you're sick, that's another story: If you have anything more serious than a mild head cold, you may be better off resting or meditating than exercising aerobically.)

Initially, you may want to monitor your physical activity in an exercise diary (see the Appendix) so that you can see connections between what you're doing and how you're feeling while you're exercising and afterwards. Does your body feel recharged or exhausted? Does exercise clear your mind of worries? Are negative statements—"I'm so slow" or "I'd rather be vegging in front of the TV"—floating through your mind as you exercise? Or are you enjoying the activities you've chosen? Jot down notes about any obstacles you encounter, what time of day you worked out, for how long, and whether you noticed any changes in your symptoms before or after exercising. Be sure to include all physical activities even if they don't qualify as formal exercise—things like walking to work or mowing the lawn, for example.

DESIGNING YOUR WORKOUT

What's the ideal exercise for PMS relief? Here are several activities that many women find helpful:

Walking

It's a great choice because you already know how to do it, and it's safe for almost everyone. In fact, most experts recommend that previously sedentary people or other deconditioned individuals begin with a walking program since it provides an easy way to start exercising while monitoring intensity and the effects of exercise. The pace and locale can also be tailored to individual differences and fitness levels. To spice it up, you can pump your arms vigorously—in a power walking style—to bring your heart rate up. You can make it social by inviting a friend to join you. You can vary the scenery by taking to the hills or the shore now and then. Or, you can do a walking meditation by silently repeating a mantra or prayer and focusing on the sensations in your body as you stride.

Jogging

It's more physically demanding than walking—which is why it burns more calories per minute—so it's prudent to initially intersperse walking and jogging if you want to take up jogging. After a warm-up period, jog for one minute then walk for the same amount of time; increase the lengths of these bouts gradually. As you become stronger, the amount of time you can safely spend jogging will increase. Always finish a jog by walking for a few minutes then stretching.

Aerobics classes

Many women find that the group experience of aerobics classes increases their motivation to exercise. And these days, there are plenty of aerobics classes to choose from—high- or low-impact, step aerobics, water aerobics, funk and hip-hop classes, boxing aerobics, and more. Most classes last about an hour and include warm-up, aerobic, and cool-down components. For those who find walking or jogging too monotonous, aerobics classes offer music, a variety of routines, and social interaction. (You can also supplement classes with aerobics videos at home.)

Bicycling

Whether you use a stationary bike or cycle in the great outdoors, bicycling is an ideal aerobic choice for those who can't stand the relentless pounding or the steady pace of jogging. If you cycle indoors, you can combine it with reading, listening to music, or watching TV to make it more enjoyable. If you cycle outside, you can enjoy the scenery and the fresh air—and cover more ground than you could on foot.

Swimming

Many women find that being immersed in water is soothing and relaxing and can be helpful for relieving symptoms of PMS, whether or not they swim at a fast enough pace for it to be considered aerobic. In an

Olympic-size pool, 72 laps equals one mile, and as with other forms of exercise, you'll need to gradually increase your endurance even if you're accustomed to other forms of exercise. Yes, swimming and other forms of aquatic exercise are generally easier on the body than land-based workouts—thanks to the water's natural cushioning and buoyancy—but working against the water also challenges—and hence improves—body strength because it offers 12 times the resistance of air.

Gym Machines

At gyms and health clubs, there are all sorts of high-tech machines to choose from these days—treadmills, stationary bicycles (including the upright, recumbent, and arm-handle varieties), stair-climbers, elliptical machines, cross-country skiers, rowing machines, and climbing machines, to name a few. But exercising in place—and in the same setting, day after day—can become monotonous so it's a good idea to vary your routine by using different machines on different days or creating your own circuit program (in which you do short spurts on one machine then move on to another and so on). Fortunately, many of these machines offer the advantage of allowing you to read or listen to music while you work out.

▪ *Cautionary Measures* ▪

If you experience any of the following symptoms while exercising, stop and seek medical advice:

- Chest, arm, or joint pain
- Unusual shortness of breath
- Irregular heartbeat
- Dizziness, lightheadedness, or fainting
- Nausea or vomiting
- Muscle or joint problems that persist
- Prolonged fatigue
- Unexplained changes in exercise tolerance

These could suggest an underlying medical problem that warrants attention.

Above all, the key is to find the form of exercise that creates the desired effect in you. If you want to ease moderate anxiety and tension, performing vigorous exercise—such as 45 minutes of jogging or an hour of cycling or swimming—three to five times per week across the menstrual cycle can help. But during the premenstrual week, certain forms of high-energy activities—like Spinning or kick-boxing, for example—can make some women feel more revved up, which isn't what you want if your premenstrual symptoms tend to rank high in tension, irritability, or mood swings. In that case, you might be better off doing a mini-workout with a shorter jog or swim, or opting for yoga, stretching, or other relaxing exercises during the premenstrual week. After all, if you already feel as though you're bouncing off the walls emotionally or your head is pounding with a premenstrual headache, why compound those sensations with highly charged forms of exercise?

On the other hand, if fatigue, the blues, or insomnia tend to bother you most premenstrually, then high-energy activities may be just what you need to relieve these symptoms and rejuvenate your spirits. If you are having trouble sleeping, consider exercising early in the day or before 2 or 3 P.M. when cortisol levels naturally start to decline and begin to shift into nighttime rhythms.

WORKING OUT THE KINKS

When you feel stiff, tense, and physically out of sorts premenstrually, you need to coax your muscles into releasing tension and remembering how to relax. The best way to do this is with a well designed stretching routine that will boost circulation, ease muscle tension and stiffness, and quiet a racing mind. The exercises that follow can help revive taut and tired muscles from head to toe, leaving you feeling relaxed and refreshed. Best of all, this routine can be done anytime—first thing in the morning, before or after a workout, midday at your desk, or before turning in for the night—and almost anyplace. Remember to do these slowly and to breathe fully as you do these stretches; pay attention to any tight spots and stop and breathe into them before moving on to the next stretch. With all of these moves, be sure to stretch to the point of gentle tension; never push a stretch or bounce into it.

- **Start by taking a full, deep breath.** Place your hands on your belly and inhale, expanding your belly and pushing it forward as you fill up with air. Exhale slowly, tightening your abdominal muscles as you push the air out.

- **Do shoulder rolls.** With your arms relaxed at your sides, lift your shoulders toward your ears and slowly roll them forward, down, back, and up again in a series of five smooth circles. Then, reverse the roll by lifting your shoulders then rolling them back toward your shoulder blades, down, forward, and up again in a series of five smooth circles.

- **Roll your head around.** Stand with your arms relaxed by your sides and your shoulders back and relaxed. Slowly bend your head forward, relaxing the back of your neck, then gently rotate your head to the left side so that your left ear is over your left shoulder. Then, roll your head forward again and over to the right side, so that your right ear is over your right shoulder. Do four complete swings in each direction. (Note: Skip this exercise if you have a neck injury or disk problem.)

- **Perform arm circles.** In a standing position, hold your arms straight out to your sides with your elbows straight and your wrists bent so that your palms are up (pretend you're impersonating a traffic cop). Keep your arms in this position and slowly rotate them forward in a large circular motion so that you're moving them from the shoulders. Do four large circles in this direction then do four more in the reverse direction.

- **Touch your shoulder blades together.** Stand up and bring both elbows up and out to the side almost like wings, while keeping your hands in front of your chest. Keeping your head and neck in their proper alignment, try to squeeze your shoulder blades together behind you. Hold this position for 15 seconds then relax.

- **Reach for the sky.** From a standing position, with your shoulders down and your head facing forward, reach your hands overhead, straight up toward the sky with your palms facing each other. Spread your fingers and reach a little higher. Hold this position for 15 seconds then relax.

- **Stretch your sides.** Stand with your feet slightly wider than hip-width apart and place your hands overhead with your palms together. Bend gently to the right and hold this position for several seconds then return to standing. Repeat to the left side. Do this four times on each side.

- **Do side twists.** Stand with your feet a few inches apart, bend your elbows, and place your hands in front of your chest, grasping one hand with the other. (Your elbows and forearms should be parallel to the floor.) Breathe in, as you lengthen your spine, and exhale as you twist slowly to the right, leading with the right elbow. Twist as far as you can comfortably go, feeling the stretch all along your back. Breathe in again and return to the starting position. Repeat to the left side. Do three of these in each direction.

- **Bend to the floor.** Stand tall with your feet parallel, about shoulder-width apart, and your hands relaxed at your sides. Take a few deep breaths then bend forward from the hips, as far as you can, dropping your hands toward the floor in front of you. Let your head hang and hold this position for several seconds. Then slowly return to a standing position, bending your knees as you rise and feeling your spine uncurl vertebrae by vertebrae.

- **Flex your hip muscles.** While in a standing position, bend your knees slightly and gently rock your pelvis forward and back several times. Then, stand up straight, take a big step back with your left foot, keeping your feet hip-width apart, and bend your right knee: Keep your back straight but tilt your pelvis forward so that you feel a stretch along your upper left thigh and hip area. Hold this position for 30 seconds then repeat with the other side.

- **Stretch your thigh muscles.** First, stand up and place your feet hip-width apart. Move your right foot forward until your right heel is in line with your left toes, with your feet still hip-width apart (there should be a considerable space between your feet). Bend your left knee, keeping your right leg straight, and then bend forward at the waist, keeping your back flat. You should feel the stretch in your right hamstring (the muscle along the back of your thigh). Hold this position for 20 seconds then return to standing.

Next, to stretch the quadriceps (the muscle along the front of your thigh), stand on the floor and put your weight on your left foot. Bend your right knee and with your right hand, pull the right heel straight back toward your buttocks. (You can hold on to a wall with your left hand for balance, if need be.) Hold for five seconds then release. Repeat both exercises on the left side.

- **Extend your calves.** Stand a few feet away from a wall and lean forward, placing your hands against the wall for support. Bring your right leg forward, bending your knee and placing your foot flat on the floor. Lean toward the wall until you feel a good stretch in your left calf muscle. Hold this position for five to ten seconds. Switch sides.

- **Draw ankle circles.** Sit on the floor with your legs extended in front of you and your hands on the floor by your hips. Flex your right foot and slowly make five clockwise circles in the air then relax. Repeat with the left foot. Then, flex your right foot again and make five circles in a counterclockwise direction. Repeat with the left foot.

THE SOOTHING POWER OF YOGA

Many women find it difficult to continue engaging in aerobic exercise during the premenstrual phase due to breast tenderness, abdominal bloating, or cyclical headaches. If this is true for you, there's no need to shirk your workout entirely: Simply choose a less intense, less jarring form of exercise. One of the easiest and most effective ways to modify an exercise regimen is to add yoga, an ancient Indian exercise system that is based on the belief that the body and breath are intimately connected with the mind. By controlling your breathing and holding the body in steady poses or "asanas," the practice of yoga can put your body into a state of harmony.

Yoga can ease muscle tension, improve the function of internal organs, and enhance the flexibility of the joints, ligaments, and muscles. What's more, it can relieve stress, anxiety, irritability, and fatigue—and help you reclaim a sense of well-being. There are four central elements to the practice of yoga: proper breathing, poses, relaxation, and meditation. Each pose is performed slowly, with gentle, fluid movements and proper breathing techniques. This draws vital energy into your body, calming your muscles and organs, and allowing you to release stress, fatigue, and toxic thoughts. Yoga poses can be rejuvenating, too, and reduce feelings of depression and lethargy.

These days, yoga is everywhere. You can find yoga classes at local colleges and community centers, at health clubs and gyms, or at specialized yoga centers. Some good yoga videotapes and books are available, as well. (You'll find a list in the resources section of the Appendix.) Fortunately, you can practice yoga in the privacy of your home, at a time that suits you. After all, you don't need any fancy equipment; nor do you need a special setting. All you need is an open space in a well-lit, comfortably heated room that's free of disturbances. Wear loose, comfortable clothing so that your movements won't be restricted. Spread a mat, towel or soft blanket over the floor or carpet for extra comfort. Wait at least an hour and a half after a meal to perform yoga.

TAKING THE MODERATE COURSE

While many experts recommend exercising five or more times per week, this isn't always feasible, as you well know. The last thing you want to do is to set yourself up for another source of stress—feeling guilty about not exercising as much as you "should." The reality is, despite their best intentions, many women just can't carve out the time to work out on a daily basis or to fit more than one or two types of exercise into their busy lives. That's why it's important to be practical about what you can do. To start, it may make sense to begin with 20 minutes of walking or another gentle form of exercise three times a week—or to set aside five to ten minutes several days per week for stretching or yoga moves.

That's a lesson Paula, 36, an accountant, learned the hard way. "I used to try to exercise every day and for too long," she explains. "My muscles hurt and felt fatigued all the time. And I'd feel like a failure when I didn't exercise daily." While participating in the UCSF program, she began to set more reasonable exercise-related goals and to look for ways to support those goals. "I started out slowly this time and I asked my husband and my kids to help me keep my scheduled time for exercise," she says. "My friends help, too, by motivating me to exercise when I'm not feeling energetic."

Paula started doing yoga once a week as well as stretching exercises at home. Gradually, she added a low-impact aerobics class three times a week and, within six months, she'd increased her yoga sessions to three times per week. "Doing this step by step made so much of a difference; this way, I didn't feel so overwhelmed," she says. "With the combination of diet changes, yoga, and aerobics, I feel so much better and my PMS is much less severe than it used to be."

Time constraints aside, remember: It's better to do a short stint of some form of physical activity than not to do anything at all. Even mundane tasks—like walking the dog, taking the stairs, or gardening—count when it comes to burning calories and improving mood and physical fitness. In fact, many health organizations have begun to emphasize the benefits of cumulative exercise throughout the day. At the very least, it will give you a chance to take a break from what you're doing, to shift gears and recoup your spirits.

When you are exercising optimally, you will feel energized and content, not worn out. You will feel a sense of accomplishment about what you're doing and perhaps a sense of empowerment, a can-do spirit as a result of including more movement in your life. As you continue to exercise, your endurance level is likely to increase and you won't feel as sore after a workout as you might have initially. Just be sure to give yourself plenty of time to increase the duration, frequency, or intensity of your workouts gradually. There's no race when it comes to exercising for PMS relief. The goal here is to help yourself feel better all month long, not to win a marathon.

YOUR ASSIGNMENT:

Spend a little time thinking about the goals you'd like to set for incorporating more exercise and physical activity into your life. To stimulate ideas, answer the following questions:

□ Do you prefer moderate physical activity, vigorous exercise, strength-training, or flexibility-enhancing routines? Which specific types of activities appeal to you in these areas?

□ How would you describe your attitude toward exercise? If you dislike it, try to pinpoint why: Is it because exercise feels like work, not play? Is it because you don't feel good about yourself when you go to the gym?

☐ What specific changes are you willing to make in your exercise regimen? What are your fitness-related goals?

☐ Have you tried to make similar changes to your exercise life in the past? If so, what were the results and how did you feel while trying to make those changes?

☐ List as many concrete actions and ideas as you can (joining a gym, finding an exercise buddy, buying an exercise video, and so on) for meeting your exercise goals.

☐ What might hinder you from reaching your goals (time constraints, inclement weather, lack of childcare, negative expectations, and the like)? How will you deal with those obstacles?

☐ Who will you ask to help or support you in achieving your goals?

6

The Role of Relaxation

At first blush, it may appear to be a bit of a chicken-and-egg question: Does stress cause PMS or does PMS cause stress? The truth is, stress does not cause PMS per se, but research does suggest that stressful events can exacerbate premenstrual symptoms. This is due, in large measure, to the fact that many of the neuroendocrine secretions that are associated with the human stress response are also associated with aggravating PMS. On the other hand, there's no question that premenstrual symptoms can be stressful in their own right. Who would dispute that it can be upsetting, frustrating, even maddening to experience sudden flashes of physical discomfort or mood changes for as much as half of each month? But dealing with the combination of stress and premenstrual symptoms can be like wrestling with a double-edged sword—precarious, to say the least!— which is why it's important for any woman who experiences PMS to practice stress-management strategies.

After all, stress can have far-reaching effects on your body and mind. A woman's response to stressful events can activate some body systems and hormone-secreting glands while shutting down other systems in the brain and body. In the anatomy of the stress response, there are three primary stages that affect mind and body—the on-alert stage, the stress preparation stage, and the action stage. In the on-alert stage, your brain registers the stress as a threat by evaluating relevant information that's available; this initial information is then amplified with emotional arousal and an instantaneous heightening of all the senses, almost like the internal flashing of a red-alert warning light.

Next, the body prepares for action—to fight or flee, in primitive terms—and the brain's messengers, particularly neurotransmitters and hormones, are released into the bloodstream; at the same time, electrical impulses are fired through the nervous systems to activate the whole body to deal with the perceived threat. Acute stress as well as everyday hassles can spark the release of adrenaline, which increases your heart rate and respiratory rate, raises blood pressure, increases blood sugar levels, and boosts alertness. Over time, these repeated physiological changes can have detrimental effects on your heart and arteries, digestion, skin, reproductive function, immune function, and other bodily systems.

In the third stage of the stress response, which takes place if the body decides to take action or if the stress continues, the hormones cortisol and DHEA (dehydroepiandrosterone) are secreted throughout the day and night to help your body function. During the stress response, secretion of aldosterone, antidiuretic hormone, and glucocorticoids are also increased. When the brain senses prolonged stress, even more of these hormones are secreted, which upsets the body's homeostasis or balance and magnifies your behavioral and symptomatic responses to stress.

Regardless of what triggers it, we've all experienced the stress response: We know it when it happens because our hearts beat faster. Our muscles tense. We breathe harder. We might break out in a light sweat. And we feel as though we're on red-alert status. All of these physiological responses were incredibly useful back in the ages when man (or woman) had to fend off wild animals, but they're less helpful as we try to cope with the psychological sources of stress that are abundant in today's world. A surge of adrenaline and a faster heart rate are not going to help you figure out how to pay your bills when you're broke, for example. And yet it doesn't seem to matter whether the threat to which the body is responding is psychological or physical, real or imagined (based on fear); the body will respond the same way and will manifest the same symptoms.

While most of us know what kinds of situations typically cause our shoulders to tense or our ire to boil, we may not always be as aware of the heavy toll these explosive moments exact on our physical and psychological health. We may not realize, for example, that subtle metabolic and psychological processes are occurring inside us, processes that can lead to health problems—from headaches and irregular periods to digestive distress and heart palpitations to more frequent infections—if the stress response is triggered repeatedly. And we may not realize that high levels of stress hormones such as adrenaline could be fueling anxiety. Whether we're dealing with personal conflicts, a mistake made at work, waiting in a traffic jam, or worrying about paying for a child's education, the stress response generates physical reactions that don't necessarily disappear once the concerns drift out of our minds. The body may keep working at a higher intensity, and each subsequently stressful situation is likely to provoke even more intense emotions. When combined with the increased emotional sensitivity that often characterizes the premenstrual phase of the menstrual cycle, these stress-induced feelings are likely to become intensified, which can, in turn, exacerbate premenstrual symptoms.

Isabelle, 38, a graphic designer and a mother of a preschool-aged child, juggles a highly demanding workload, a busy family life, an active exercise schedule, and numerous volunteer commitments. She manages to keep her life running fairly efficiently most of the time but meeting deadlines and staying on an even emotional keel become more of a struggle premenstrually. "When I used to just get bloating and breast tenderness before my period, that didn't bother me so much," she explains. "But in the last few years, I've started experiencing mood changes that can drive me around the bend. Suddenly all of the stress in my life becomes magnified to the nth degree and I start overreacting to little things—my son spilling his orange juice, the dog barking excessively, messiness in the house. I get this wired, agitated feeling that seems to prime me to react to even small stuff that's just not worth sweating. And that often makes me feel worse physically, too."

Studies have found that women with premenstrual symptoms often experience increased physiological arousal—including elevated heart rate and respiratory rate, increased muscle tension and sweating— that's consistent with a stress response. Other research has found that the stress response may further disrupt the cyclical balancing act between estrogen and progesterone. In addition, stress hormones such as adrenaline and cortisol have been found to be elevated in women with PMS compared to women without PMS, and these higher stress-hormone levels seem to be related to the severity of premenstrual mood changes.

A CYCLE OF REACTIVITY

Of course, anticipating PMS can be a source of stress in its own right. Women come to dread it and brace themselves for its arrival, which puts their brains and bodies on alert status. Various emotions can strengthen a memory but negative ones seem to make an indelible impression on the brain. This process is enhanced when the memory reinforces a particular image you have of yourself, whether it's that you're poor at math or you struggle with PMS. It appears that the level of activity in the part of the brain called the amygdala (which is located close to the hypothalamus which regulates menstrual cycle hormones) predicts how well you will remember bombing on a math test or yelling at your child when you have PMS. When you experience a threatening event or you anticipate the negative emotions that are associated with recurring PMS, amygdala activity increases and helps to sustain the negative perceptions. Stress hormones also come into play and strengthen the neuronal circuit that embodies a distressing memory.

In addition, recent research at the National Institute of Mental Health has demonstrated how a regularly recurring source of stress can activate the physiological stress response. Basically, there is a kindling effect, similar to the way cocaine arouses the brain: After repeated experiences, very small amounts of the same stimulus can subsequently activate the same level of arousal. Even thinking about ingesting cocaine—or experiencing PMS, in this case—will stimulate the arousal response.

Yet studies have also found that many women claim their premenstrual symptoms precipitated stressful experiences such as relationship conflicts or increased sensitivity to their impact. In a study at the University of Washington, women with PMS and PMM symptom patterns reported more sources of stress and higher stress levels than women with a low severity pattern did; the former groups also reported that their stress levels typically increased premenstrually. But only the women who had the classic PMS pattern had higher levels of adrenaline, which is associated with physical arousal and turmoil symptoms. In considering which came first, premenstrual symptoms or stress, these researchers found a reciprocal relationship: that perceived stress often precedes premenstrual symptoms but that symptoms can also occur before stress. It may be that the two factors fuel each other, making a woman increasingly reactive—physically, emotionally, and behaviorally—to what's happening in her environment.

Indeed, psychologist Karen Blechman, Ph.D., of the University of Colorado in Boulder, has proposed a "danger-signal" theory of PMS in which a woman who has been socialized to expect menstruation to be negative searches for signals that menstrual bleeding will soon begin. This premenstrual vigilance results in general physiologic arousal and negative mood, which, in turn, reduce a woman's tolerance for stress and makes her premenstrual changes more pronounced. When a woman starts looking, month after month, for premenstrual symptoms as a sign that her period will soon arrive, this eternal vigilance can reinforce feelings of anxiety, depression, and distress, as well as maladaptive coping behaviors such as overeating. What's more, this state of hypervigilance can activate the fight-or-flight response, aggravating her premenstrual symptoms further and increasing her risk of stress-related illness. Making matters worse, many women with PMS use strategies, such as stepping up their exercise routines or packing their schedules with extra activities to stay busy, that may actually increase their stress. It can all add up to an endless loop of premenstrual stress and symptoms.

MAKING STRESS LESS DISTRESSING

One thing is absolutely certain: Just as stress management is now considered a vital part of leading a healthy lifestyle, the same is true when it comes to managing PMS. After all, stress appears to be an immutable fact of modern life and while you can't eliminate it, you can modify your perception of stressful events as well as your reaction to them. (You'll learn more about how to alter your mindset in the next chapter.) You can also use relaxation strategies on a regular basis to prevent stress from wearing you down physically or tearing you up emotionally.

The first step in learning any stress management technique usually involves learning how to breathe slowly and rhythmically. Of course, proper breathing habits are always important for good physical and mental health: When an insufficient amount of fresh air reaches your lungs, your blood is not properly oxygenated, waste products are not removed efficiently, digestion is hampered, and organs and tissues are undernourished. Plus, it becomes that much harder to cope with anxiety, fatigue, and depression.

In my research, we found that many women with PMS have slightly higher than normal levels of carbon dioxide and lower levels of oxygen in their blood. And we couldn't figure out why. As we interviewed the women, it became apparent that they were breathing shallowly, which is almost like hyperventilating and makes symptoms of anxiety worse. The solution is to practice abdominal breathing. Lean slightly forward, breathe in through your nose, pushing out your abdomen, then breathe out through your mouth (place your hands on your belly to see if you're doing it right). Practice this for a few minutes five times per day, and soon it will come naturally.

--- ■ *Breathing 101* ■ ---

Proper breathing habits are essential for good mental and physical health. They can also be antidotes to stress and fatigue, especially when combined with stretching or relaxation exercises. The truth is, you can vary your breathing pattern to achieve specific effects, whether you crave relaxation or rejuvenation. Here are four techniques to help you breathe easier:

- **Deep Breathing:** Lie down on the floor and bend your knees so that your feet are flat on the floor. Place one hand on your abdomen and one hand on your chest. Inhale slowly and deeply through your nostrils, allowing air to fill up your abdomen, causing your hand to rise. Hold the breath for a second then slowly exhale through your mouth, making a quiet *whooshing* sound like the wind as you blow the air out and cause your abdomen to empty. Practice this for three to five minutes at a stretch.
- **Relaxing Sigh:** Because a sigh naturally releases a bit of tension, you can use this to your advantage. Sit or stand up straight and sigh deeply,

making a sound of deep relief as the air rushes out of your lungs. Then, just let the air come back in naturally. Repeat this eight to 12 times, on an as-needed basis.

- **The Natural Breath:** It's a matter of trying to breathe like a baby—in a natural manner. Sit or stand up straight and breathe in through your nose. As you inhale, start by filling the lower section of your lungs; your diaphragm will push your abdomen out to make room for the air. Next, fill the middle part of your lungs, as your lower ribs and chest move slightly forward to accommodate the air. Finally, fill the upper part of your lungs, as you raise your chest slightly. Try to practice these three steps in one smooth, continuous inhalation. Hold your breath for a second then exhale slowly, pulling your abdomen in slightly as the lungs empty.

- **Rejuvenating Breath:** When you feel low on energy, this exercise will stimulate your breathing and circulation. Stand up straight with your hands by your sides. Inhale slowly in the "natural breath" pattern described above, and as you do this, raise your arms toward the ceiling and stretch. Exhale and relax, lowering your arms back to your sides. Repeat this several times until you feel the stimulating effects.

Few studies have explored the direct effects of stress management on PMS, although a study at Harvard Medical School examined the use of the relaxation response—eliciting a state of profound, almost meditative calm—for the treatment of PMS and found a 58 percent reduction in physical and emotional symptoms over five months. In my research, almost all of the women with PMS used one or more relaxation techniques. Over the long-term about one-third used relaxation techniques on a daily basis, and over half of the women used them on an as-needed basis. At first, many women struggled with quieting their minds before they could get their bodies to relax. Adding cognitive strategies, which you'll read about in the next chapter, helped them reduce obsessive or worrisome thoughts so that they could focus more fully on easing tension in their bodies and minds.

There are many different ways to elicit the relaxation response, including yoga, exercise, meditation, progressive muscle relaxation, autogenic training, imagery, and self-hypnosis, among others. All of these can be somewhat slow to master but you will feel some benefits from even your first attempts. Try not to be impatient: It's impossible to reverse years of habit with a single effort to relax. But if you set aside at least 15 minutes each day to practice these techniques, you'll become adept at eliciting the relaxation response within ten to 14 days. Once you have mastered the basic techniques of inducing relaxation, you can use them almost anywhere—at home or at work, in your car or on a crowded bus, at your in-laws' house, or on a lengthy line at the grocery store—probably without even closing your eyes. The only way to discover which strategy is right for you is to experiment with various techniques and see how they feel. Be sure to wear loose, comfortable clothing as you do these. You'll find basic instructions below but many of these techniques can also be learned with the aid of audio- or videotapes, if you crave more detailed instruction.

Progressive muscle relaxation:

Developed in the 1920's by an American psychologist named Edmund Jacobsen, progressive muscle relaxation (PMR) is a technique that focuses the mind on systematically tensing and relaxing various groups of muscles from head to toe. The goal is to release muscle tension throughout the body. An additional benefit is that the technique fosters body awareness: While tightening then releasing various muscles, you'll enhance your awareness of tense versus relaxed body states. As you become increasingly skilled in this technique, you'll be able to do a quick scan of your body for tension and relax the body more quickly simply with deep breathing.

How to do it:

Sit or lie down in a warm, quiet place. If you'll be sitting, use a cushioned chair that supports your back and neck, if possible, and place your hands on your lap. If you'll be lying down, place a cushion or pillow under your head and knees and let your hands and arms rest by your side or on your stomach. When you feel comfortable, take a few deep breaths, exhaling in a gentle sigh. Start by making a fist with your right hand, tensing the muscles in your forearm as well. Hold this position for five seconds then release it, relaxing the muscles in your hand and forearm. Next, tense the muscles in your right upper arm by bending your elbow, bringing your hand toward your shoulder; hold for five seconds then relax. Repeat these moves with your left hand and arm.

Then, focus on your face. Raise your eyebrows toward the top of your crown, wrinkling your forehead; hold for five seconds then relax. Next, squint your eyes and wrinkle your nose for five seconds then release. Then, purse your lips, pushing them out in an exaggerated kiss, hold this for five seconds, then open your lips, clench your teeth, and make a wide smile. Hold for five seconds then relax.

Your shoulders, back, and trunk are next: Bring your shoulders up toward your ears, hold for five seconds, then release. Now, breathe deeply and try to touch your shoulder blades behind you; hold for five seconds then release. Next, suck in your abdomen, as if you were trying to squeeze into a pair of tight jeans; hold for five seconds, then release. Tense both buttock muscles; hold for five seconds, then release.

Moving down to the legs, push your right foot against the floor (if you're sitting) or raise your right leg about six inches from the floor (if you're lying down), and tense the muscles in your right thigh; hold this for five seconds then relax. To tense your right calf muscle, point your toes and lift your heel up; hold for five seconds then release. Next, point your toes again for five seconds, flex your right foot at the ankle for five seconds, then relax. Repeat these moves on the left side.

At the end of these exercises, breathe in deeply and wiggle your fingers and toes to restimulate circulation. Rest in this position for a few minutes, then stand up slowly, stretching your arms and shaking your hands and feet a few more times before getting on with your day (or evening).

Shortened muscle relaxation:
After you have mastered the PMR exercise—it takes about two weeks of daily practice—you may want to use a shorter version that takes only five to ten minutes each day.

How to do it:
After getting into a comfortable position, start with slow, deep breaths: Breathe in so that the air you inhale pushes your abdomen out; take each breath at a rhythm that feels right to you and exhale with a sigh, imagining the tension is flowing out of your body as you release each breath. Then, stretch your shoulders and neck by doing slow head rolls.

Bend both elbows and point them toward the ceiling, tensing the hands (by making fists), forearms, and upper arms. Hold for five to ten seconds then relax. Next, simultaneously raise your eyebrows, squint your eyes, wrinkle your nose, and purse your lips into an exaggerated kiss; hold for five to ten seconds then release. For your neck and upper back, stretch your head away from your shoulders, clench your teeth and make a wide smile, and try to touch your shoulder blades together behind you; hold this position for five to ten seconds then release.

Next, suck in your abdomen and tighten your buttocks simultaneously; hold for five to ten seconds then relax. And, finally, if you're lying down, raise both legs about six inches from the floor, flexing your feet toward your head; if you're sitting, press your feet against the floor then extend both legs, alternately pointing your toes and bending your ankles and flexing your feet—do these moves for five to ten seconds then relax.

Autogenic training:
In this technique, which is similar to progressive muscle relaxation, sensory cues are used to relax your muscles from head to toe. The first step is to focus on the powers of mental suggestion as you train your muscles to relax by suggesting that they are becoming warm and heavy. Autogenic training teaches your body and mind to respond quickly and effectively to your verbal commands to relax and return to a balanced state in which you feel calm and competent. To achieve the right state of relaxation, you may need to practice this daily for two weeks.

How to do it:
Choose a comfortable sitting or reclining position—following the same guidelines as with progressive muscle relaxation—then close your eyes, breathe slowly and deeply, and repeat the following commands under your breath. Repeat each one until you feel the desired result then, and only then, continue to the next one.

- "My whole body is relaxed; nothing will disturb me."
- "My arms feel heavy. My arms feel warm and heavy."
- "My legs feel heavy. My legs feel warm and heavy."

- "My neck and shoulders feel heavy. My neck and shoulders feel warm and heavy."

- "My heart is beating steadily and calmly."

- "My abdomen is feeling warm and relaxed."

- "My buttocks are feeling warm and relaxed."

- "My forehead feels cool and clear."

- "I am completely at rest. My whole body is relaxed. Each muscle is limp and relaxed. Nothing can disturb me. I am completely at rest."

- "These feelings of rest and well-being will accompany me everywhere. I will gain confidence and strength from them. I will feel refreshed, just like after a deep and peaceful sleep."

Now, breathe deeply. Become aware of how your body feels, stretch, then open your eyes. If you continue to feel tension in any particular area, you can add more sensory language to enhance relaxation in that part of the body.

Meditation:
Various forms of meditation—Transcendental Meditation, mindfulness meditation, moving meditation, and so on—can have a calming effect on the mind and body, producing a full relaxation response. This is achieved by focusing your attention and harnessing the power of the mind to induce a state of inner peace and tranquility. Research has found that meditation's ability to quiet—or reverse—the stress response has physical benefits, too, such as reducing the severity of arthritis, asthma, chronic pain, diabetes, gastrointestinal disorders, hot flashes, hypertension, and migraine headaches. Several studies have also reported that people who receive meditation instruction experience less pain and anxiety from various causes and use less medication in treating these symptoms. Meditation can also increase psychological insight by quieting and clearing mental chaos; this helps clear away distorted perceptions of the world, allowing lucid, astute observations to emerge in the process.

How to do it:

Different forms of meditation use slightly different techniques, and many require hands-on training with an expert. Here's a method that is simple and easy to learn on your own: Sit comfortably in a position that suits you. Select a word (such as *serenity*), a sound (such as *whoosh*) or a phrase (you're on your own with this one) that appeals to you for your mantra. Close your eyes, relax the muscles throughout your body, and breathe slowly and naturally, repeating your mantra silently each time you exhale. Try not to examine or criticize how well you're doing with your meditation; if other thoughts enter your mind, picture them as surrounded by a bubble and let the bubble drift slowly up to the sky while you return to focusing on your mantra. Or, you can picture yourself placing your worries in a box and putting it on a train that's leaving the station. (This "letting go" technique is based largely on Buddhist philosophy.) Continue this for about 20 minutes (or even ten minutes if that's all you can spare) then open your eyes. Sit and relax for a few minutes longer before going about your business.

As simple as meditation sounds, it's not always easy to do. You'll need to practice self-discipline in order to avoid reacting to the many stimuli around you as well as in your mind and body as you try to concentrate. When practiced regularly, however, meditation does get easier. In my research, many women found that practicing early in the morning was easier than later in the day, perhaps because their days weren't yet full of distractions. After about two weeks of daily practice, you'll probably notice how much easier it is to slip into a meditative, relaxed state. As an added benefit, over time, you are likely to find that solutions to problems you've been worrying about will often enter your mind during meditation.

SHORTCUTS TO SELF-SOOTHING

There are a few other quick, calming strategies you can use to help yourself de-stress wherever you go. If you find yourself tensing up in a social situation, excuse yourself for a few minutes and find a quiet corner (in the bathroom, if need be): Sit or lean against the wall, close your eyes, empty your mind, and concentrate on practicing deep, even breathing as you let the tension dissipate and disappear.

Sometimes, simply repeating a cue word—such as *calm*—several times to yourself, while you try to recall the feeling of being calm and relaxed, can help you return to that state. Because most of us stop breathing fully when we feel stressed or anxious, practicing breath control in the form of deep, regular abdominal breathing can help, too. Whether you're stuck in traffic or in the midst of a family squabble, concentrate on taking two to three deep belly breaths then continue breathing from your belly in a more natural rhythm. If you have trouble remembering to breathe fully during stressful times, post a reminder—a note that reads "Breathe!"—on your computer, the phone, your dashboard, or wherever you need it.

Another technique that can help decrease tension in a pinch is to count backward as you consciously relax each body part. Try to relax from top to bottom, inside and out, as you count slowly in this fashion: 10-Head, 9-Face, 8-Neck, 7-Upper back, 6-Arms, 5-Lower back, 4-Stomach, 3-Buttocks, 2-Legs, and 1-Inner tension. Afterwards, take two or three deep, cleansing breaths and try to maintain your newly relaxed state.

GETTING AWAY FROM IT ALL MENTALLY

Women who have crowded schedules often have overcrowded minds, too. With too many things to do, remember, and keep track of, it's no wonder their concentration abilities can become weak and fragmented. There's no question that it can be incredibly frustrating to have your mind wander when you're trying to train your attention, concentration, and creativity on a particular task or trying to stay in control of a busy schedule and you're feeling exhausted premenstrually.

What women need to do, in these instances, is take a mental mini-vacation, using imagery, to recharge their emotional and cognitive batteries. The use of imagery is not only a powerful stress-reduction strategy but when combined with relaxation or meditation techniques, it can be a potent physical and mental coping skill that can result in lowered blood pressure, decreased muscle tension, and a relaxation of brain waves. It can also help you put your best foot forward in specific situations: Many athletes, for example, use imagery—in which they might see themselves performing well under pressure or winning a race—as part of their training programs. You can do the same. After all, imagery and visualization techniques are close cousins to something we all naturally do throughout our lives—daydream. The difference is, imagery is more focused or guided and usually more intense than daydreaming is.

By using imagery, you can recondition your mind and body to better deal with the inevitable stress of a busy life and the cyclical stress of PMS. It can also help you ease feelings of agitation and nervousness, boost low energy, relieve boredom or the blues, and even bolster your self-confidence. The key is to develop a personalized scenario that appeals to you. You'll need a pad of paper or your PMS notebook for this exercise. The first step is to note what you hope the mental mini-vacation will help you achieve: The goal could be to calm feelings of anxiety, agitation, and turmoil; it might be to rejuvenate feelings of low energy, depression, and fatigue; or, it could be to find comfort and a sense of security when you're feeling shaky and short on self-confidence. Then, write down a description of a setting, place, person, or sensory experience—whether it comes from your memory or your imagination—that would help you change the way you're feeling if you were experiencing that scenario right now. Try to be as free, creative, and inspired as possible—this is for your eyes and imagination only!

Here are some examples of what various mental mini-vacations might look like:

- **A calming mental mini-vacation:** Perhaps you see yourself on a sailboat on an open sea with a gentle wind ruffling your hair and the sails. Or perhaps you envision yourself in a lush, green meadow, having a pleasant picnic with your family. To relieve feelings of nervousness and agitation, the right mental mini-vacation will be one that you associate with feelings of serenity, peace, and calm.

- **A rejuvenating mental mini-vacation:** For some women, it might be galloping on horseback along the shore or skiing down a steep mountain at an exhilarating speed. For others, it might be imagining an erotic sexual fantasy. To relieve feelings of malaise, fatigue, or depression, conjure up your own personalized image of whatever makes you feel pumped up, motivated, or euphoric.

- **A comforting, reassuring mental mini-vacation:** Whether it's snuggling up with a fluffy comforter in front of a glowing fire or basking in the sun's warm rays on a pristine beach, the image you bring to mind should evoke feelings of comfort, reassurance, security, and safety. This can help relieve feelings of insecurity or anxiety, a crisis of confidence, or other unsettling feelings.

After you've written down the scenarios that appeal to you in each area, slowly read them out loud, trying to use the appropriate feeling and tone in your voice. If you'd like to, record yourself reading the scenario, putting yourself in the picture ("I am sitting in a fragrant, green park, holding hands with the love of my life . . ." or "I am biking down a steep hill, taking curves at breakneck speed . . ."). Don't worry about delivering your presentation flawlessly; the purpose of recording this is simply to talk the imagery into your head.

Now, get into a relaxed position—sitting in a comfortable chair or lying down on a soft surface—and listen to your first scenario on tape or recount it back to yourself. Breathe slowly and rhythmically and use the relaxation techniques that you have already mastered, while concentrating on the feeling—whether it's calm, rejuvenation, or comfort—that you intended to create with your mental mini-vacation. Continue this for five to ten minutes, letting yourself be transported to another place or experience as this movie plays itself out in the theater of your mind.

Your choice of scenario can be determined by the nature of your stress-state at a particular time: When your energy wanes in the mid-afternoon, for example, you might want to use your revitalizing mental mini-vacation instead of going for a cup of coffee. When the pressure builds at work, you might lean back, close your eyes, and recall the imagery of a calm, serene setting. Or you might choose one over another based on what's happening in your life.

Eileen, 40, a computer programmer and mother of three children, regularly used the calming mental mini-vacation for severe PMS. But as the circumstances of her life shifted, so did her imagined mini-vacation. "Now that I am going through a lot of transitions in my life—changing jobs, going to night school, and remodeling our home—I am using the comforting one almost daily," she explains. "I feel a need for reassurance and comfort, and I notice that I feel less anxious and worried about making the right decision after I take one of these mental getaways."

You can customize your imagined mini-vacation further by combining some of the qualities of the different ones into a version that appeals to your emotional needs. "Because I often feel out-of-control premenstrually, I use a mini-vacation scenario that combines calming and comforting qualities," explains Naomi, 34, an occupational therapist. "I visualize going to a warm, peaceful place, where there's a cottage surrounded by trees, a small pond, and a hammock. I imagine lying in the hammock, feeling warm and relaxed. I feel safe there because the hammock supports me. After spending some time in that wonderful place, I always feel better. My mind feels less chaotic. My neck doesn't hurt. I feel centered and peaceful again."

Since you'll want your mental mini-vacations to provide you with an escape during stressful times, you'll want to have them fully developed long before you need them, which means that you'll need to practice them regularly. After a few weeks of practice, you will find that your mind will elicit a conditioned reaction at the very thought of a particular scenario. The first few words you say to yourself will trigger a calming, revitalizing, or comforting response—a quick trip to a better state of mind.

Whether you'll be taking a mental mini-vacation or practicing a relaxation technique, try to find a time and place where you won't be disturbed. Talk to your family or roommates about this; enlist their help and support in helping you to find the time and space for this. Once you find it, treat that time as sacred, just as you would an important business appointment. Above all, try not to get discouraged if these techniques don't elicit the effect you desire right away. Remember: Your stress-related symptoms and anxieties were probably built up over years so it's unrealistic to expect to undo them within a matter of days. (And when you are especially stressed out or your PMS is at its absolute worst, it may take you much longer to relax.) As you progress with a particular relaxation exercise, you should find yourself moving from a state of tension to a sensation of release and relaxation.

Generally, it takes at least two to three weeks of regular, daily practice for a relaxation technique's sustainable benefits to kick in and for it to become a new habit for your mind and body. The good news is, once you have trained yourself to be able to relax, this will become a tool that you can pull out and use at a moment's notice, nearly anytime and anywhere. And if you do use these tools regularly, you will likely become less reactive to stress and begin to feel more empowered to handle whatever curveballs life throws your way.

<u>YOUR ASSIGNMENT</u>:

Spend a few minutes thinking about your relaxation goals and which strategies you'd like to start with. This will help you make practical choices and anticipate what might be involved. To get the ideas flowing, answer the following questions:

- ☐ Which of the relaxation strategies appeal to you most? Why? Think about your rationale and write it down.

- ☐ Have you tried similar relaxation techniques in the past? If so, are you still using them? If not, why did you stop?

- ☐ Which of the mental mini-vacations appeals to you the most? Which ones are you likely to use?

- ☐ List as many concrete actions and ideas as you can for meeting your stress-management goals.

- ☐ Now think about potential obstacles that might stand in your way (scheduling problems, time constraints, your inner critic, and the like). How will you deal with them?

- ☐ Who will you ask to help or support you in achieving your goals?

7

Giving Your Mindset a Makeover

"The mind is its own place, and in itself
Can make a heaven of Hell, a hell of Heaven."
—John Milton, *Paradise Lost*

Perception does not necessarily equal reality, and yet, for better or worse, the mind is a powerful thing when it comes to our experiences. More often than not, people's perceptions of psychological threats are inaccurate and maladaptive for their emotional and physical well-being. This is true of women with PMS, as well as those who don't suffer from this cyclical turmoil. These perceptions are simply a result of distorted ways of thinking, of self-defeating beliefs, of old scripts or worry cycles that repeat themselves endlessly in our heads, like a broken record, making us feel inadequate, insecure, and completely stressed out. What this amounts to is mental bad habits, only, in this case, women don't even realize they engage in these harmful patterns.

Women with PMS often describe their minds as racing or as feeling as though they "can't stop certain thoughts." During the premenstrual phase of their cycles, this cognitive tension can be exacerbated as irritability and other unpleasant feelings set in. As a result, many women have trouble using some of the relaxation or stress-reduction strategies when they need them most. Many women also worry that the way they behave when their PMS is flaring up could take a toll on their relationships or their careers. All of which adds up to another insidious form of stress, an internal one called cognitive stress.

How does this happen? The human brain takes in thousands of pieces of information each day and interprets them through cognitive processes, including a variety of thinking and reasoning skills. Each experience or perception goes through a cognitive deciphering process that begins with interpretation of a stimulus or piece of information through one of the senses, at which point it is evaluated in terms of its threat potential and classified as negative, neutral, or positive. If this cognitive analysis tells you that the stimulus or event is positive or benign, you may feel happy, relaxed, satisfied, or neutral. If you interpret it as negative or threatening to your physical or psychological security, then the stress response is automatically activated, sparking feelings of anxiety, anger, depression, and the numerous physiological reactions you read about in the previous chapter.

Through these experiences, we naturally develop beliefs, attitudes, values, and assumptions about others or the world that become our mind-sets. Our mind-sets typically develop over the course of our lives, and they may be influenced by our personalities, past traumas and conflicts, external events, and our families of origin. Not only does this mental programming affect how we view particular events and the world at large but it affects how we interpret our own personal experiences. And if you routinely subscribe to distorted ways of thinking, negative self-talk, or other forms of potentially toxic thinking, you are unwittingly shaping your own reality into an unpleasant experience. After all, stress results not from actual events but from your interpretation of those events. And the meaning you assign to those experiences will be largely influenced by the expectations you hold about what "should" or "should not" happen.

What's more, when you engage in cognitive distortions, you may be activating a mental and physical stress response that could end up doing damage to your body. After all, negative thoughts and constant worries keep the mind activated and the body in a constant state of tension, which can have widespread effects on the body and mind. Research has revealed, for example, that catastrophizing—viewing a relatively minor incident as serious misfortune—is associated with an increased experience of pain and with a higher risk of depression. What's more, in a recent study at the University of North Carolina,

Chapel Hill, researchers found that women with gastrointestinal disorders who engaged in catastrophic thinking had poorer health outcomes than those who didn't have this maladaptive coping style. In other words, your state of mind really can affect the state of your health quite profoundly.

The Far-Reaching Effects of Menstrual Dread

Women often learn from their mothers, sisters, friends, and the media that menstruation is something to dread or be ashamed of, and studies have found that women often associate their periods with negative moods and physical pain. Not surprisingly, this negative view has been found to influence how women interpret their own periods and premenstrual symptoms. Women who typically have premenstrual symptoms often anticipate them and perceive events that occur around the time of menstruation as more stressful. In many studies of women with PMS, 70 to 90 percent of the women can predict the onset of their periods within one to four days, which suggests a high degree of anticipation and expectation.

Moreover, many women with PMS also experience painful menstrual cramps. And women who have menstrual cycles with recurrent painful or distressing symptoms or who have hormonal alterations that are sparked by stress are vulnerable to an impairment of the body's homeostasis or natural state of balance, which can lead to a continuation of negative symptoms. Compounding these effects, if a woman has negative expectations about her period and tends to brace herself for its arrival, with all the unpleasant symptoms that accompany it, this negative mindset may enhance the severity of her premenstrual symptoms. In other words, the negative expectations can become a self-fulfilling prophecy, largely by triggering the body's stress response.

BREAKING THE CYCLE OF MENTAL BAD HABITS

The good news is, a woman can short-circuit this cascade of troubling events by changing her ways of thinking so that she doesn't come to expect the worst and so that she's not so reactive to stress. What this entails, in a nutshell, is cognitive restructuring—identifying negative thought patterns and critical assessments then correcting these distortions. But first she needs to identify how these distortions are taking shape; otherwise, she won't know how to correct them. Examples of cognitive distortions include overgeneralizing (believing in a pattern of defeat or negativity based on one bad experience); catastrophizing (seeing events as having an exaggeratedly and inappropriately negative significance); personalizing (relating negative events or other people's feelings or behavior to yourself); and negative mental filtering (discounting positive events and exaggerating negative ones). Here's a closer look at how these cognitive errors can lead to distressing feelings or behavior—and how to correct them:

Overgeneralization:
In this form of twisted thinking, one negative experience—a bad date, a traffic jam, a conflict at work—is translated into a sweeping pattern of defeat or negativity. If you make a wrong turn while driving to a friend's house, you might tell yourself, "I can't do anything right!" If your mind wanders while you're writing a report, you might silently berate yourself with: "I can't concentrate on anything when I'm premenstrual!"

How to counter this:
   Try to evaluate each event independently—rather than as part of a global pattern—and look for reasonable explanations for what happened.

Catastrophizing:
It's the Chicken Little syndrome, in which events are seen as having a negative significance or your mind magnifies the significance of a problem out of all reasonable proportion. If you hear about a friend's visit to the ER for a broken foot, your reaction might be, "Oh, how awful! That's got to be the worst thing that could happen to her." Or, if you're having trouble getting along with a supervisor at work, you might think, "That's it! My career's over. Now, I'll never get ahead."

How to counter this:
   Remind yourself that no single episode or event defines a person or relationship; nor does a single flaw or error characterize an entire project.

Personalization:
With this type of cognitive distortion, everything's about you, you, you. You might see yourself as the cause of an external event or some-one else's hurt feelings when, in fact, you couldn't possibly be responsible. If you're in charge of organizing a family reunion that winds up having to be postponed because of bad weather, you might chastise yourself, saying, "It's all my fault! I should have planned it for another time when we could have been sure about the weather." Not surprisingly, this tendency to assume responsibility or blame for something that's genuinely beyond your control is a primary source of guilt.

How to counter this:
Examine the evidence that what you're saying to yourself is true, and ask yourself what other factors—besides you—could have contributed to this situation.

Negative mental filtering:
Everything gets a dark shadow with this form of cognitive distortion because negative events are exaggerated and positive ones are discounted. One small or insignificant detail can completely eliminate all of the positive aspects of an event. If someone compliments you on a talk you gave at work, you might focus on the fact that your presentation was flawed because you had to clear your throat a couple of times.

How to counter this:
Ask yourself if you're looking at the situation in a black-or-white manner, and if so, try to find the gray zone. In other words, try to reframe the situation in a more positive or more neutral light.

Of course, these cognitive distortions aren't unique to women with PMS. But they can exacerbate the physical and emotional symptoms that women experience premenstrually. Whether it's through the power of suggestion or the sparking of the stress response, premenstrual symptoms can seem so much worse when your inner naysayer is calling attention to them in a negative way. Moreover, women are especially vulnerable to cognitive distortions during the premenstrual phase of their cycles because their self-esteem may take a downturn at this time of the month.

In my research, we have found that women with PMS experience changes in their self-esteem during the premenstrual phase, regardless of their level of stress. Women with severe PMS tend to have lower levels of self-esteem to begin with, and this lower level declines even further premenstrually. This makes sense intuitively, when you consider that mental, emotional, and bodily changes occur simultaneously during this time of the month. Besides, in our society, women are deemed to be attractive when they are considered physically or sexually desirable. A few days before the arrival of their periods, many women feel and look more tired. They experience fluid retention or acne. Their complexions may be sallow, their hair limp, their eyes puffy. In most cases, the alteration in appearance is slight, but often the woman feels a considerable loss of attractiveness, which can affect her self-esteem.

By itself, the psychological fallout of a drop in self-esteem can be harmful to a woman's well-being. When a woman is premenstrual, for example, she may experience increased anxiety and feel scared or withdrawn; or, she may feel hostile, argumentative, and aggressive. Besides being damaging to her own emotional health, both reactions will also affect the people around her and, consequently, their reaction to her. Over time, this interactive two-step can lead to a downward spiral in the quality of a woman's encounters with other people, which can, in turn, affect her self-esteem. And if she's already prone to cognitive distortions, she might develop more that are related to her PMS experiences, perhaps blaming or punishing herself for her premenstrual behavior. As a result, she might wind up adding to her bank of negative self-talk and decreasing her self-esteem further.

Naomi, the 34-year-old occupational therapist we met in Chapter Six, is all too familiar with these ripple effects. "PMS has caused a lot of strain in my relationships," she explains. "My family and friends don't want to be around me when I'm premenstrual because of my emotional reactivity and instability. Arguments erupt over little things; I say things I don't mean—then I have to apologize. When this goes on month after month, no one believes my apologies after a while. And I end up feeling like all I ever do is mess things up. And that makes me feel even more anxious and out of control."

DEALING WITH THOUGHTS THAT JUST WON'T STOP

There's no question that worry and doubt can stimulate the stress response and feelings of distress. Worrying is a form of rumination or obsession in which repetitive and intrusive trains of thought keep going around and around in your head, even though they're unrealistic, unproductive, and often anxiety-producing. Just like anything else you practice regularly, the more you worry, the more of a habit it becomes. Your internal response to these negative thoughts and worries becomes automatic, and your stress response is activated without your even being aware of it. You might feel anxious, your breathing may be shallow, and you may feel bad physically but you may not know why.

This cognitive process is likely to be exaggerated during the premenstrual phase of the menstrual cycle. In the days or weeks before your period arrives, you may feel even more sensitive to negative thoughts; or, you may be more likely to respond to stressful events with cognitive distortions. In my research, women have told me again and again that they dredge up even more worries than usual during the premenstrual phase, and that their heads feel as though they are "stuffed with too many worries, self-doubts, and negative tapes that won't stop playing." When this happens, the stress response is set into motion, and negative thoughts, cognitive distortions, and premenstrual symptoms can exacerbate this process further.

Yet, I have discovered in the course of my research that for most women these processes are outside of their awareness. They report the results of this endless cycle of thought-racing and symptoms—namely, anxiety, mental confusion, indecision, and feeling out of control—but they aren't aware of the cognitive processes that set them up for these heightened symptoms. It wasn't until they began to learn relaxation techniques such as progressive muscle relaxation or meditation that they described feelings of their "mind racing" or being "unable to stop certain thoughts." This was especially true during the premenstrual phases of their cycles when these patterns often became "obsessive" or "overwhelming."

CHANGING YOUR THINKING TO CHANGE YOUR MOOD

Cognitive therapists believe that patterns of negative thinking actually cause a person to feel anxious, depressed, or otherwise out of sorts. They also believe that by changing the way you think, you can alter how you behave and how you feel—for the better. There are two primary goals behind this approach: To help you feel better right now and to help you develop a more accurate appraisal system that will protect you from being so susceptible to distressing mood swings and interpersonal conflicts in the future. The key to changing these self-defeating patterns is to learn to identify when you're engaging in them, to stop the negative thoughts that circulate through your mind, and to correct them with a more rational, less rigid assessment. If you practice these strategies consistently, you will become less vulnerable to the downward emotional tug of PMS.

Developed in the 1960s, cognitive restructuring is a coping technique that is designed to favorably alter the current mindset from a negative, self-defeating attitude to a more positive one. It goes by several different names—cognitive appraisal, cognitive relabeling, cognitive reframing, or attitude adjustment—but the underlying premise is the same: That stress-related behaviors are initiated by mental processes—such as perceptions, interpretations, and reasoning—and that these negative patterns can be changed. The patriarch of cognitive therapy, psychologist Albert Ellis, became convinced that people could be educated to transform negative perceptions of events or irrational thoughts into more positive attitudes, which, in turn, could decrease the intensity of the stress they were experiencing.

Another psychologist, Donald Meichenbaum, developed the coping process that's now called *cognitive restructuring* as a way to modify internal scripts by tuning into the mind's conversation or self-talk. Using the concept of vaccination against infection as a model, he proposed a four-stage process to build up positive thoughts when negatively perceived events are encountered. The first step is to cultivate awareness, to identify and acknowledge negative thoughts, how they serve as sources of stress, and how they affect you emotionally. The next step is to reappraise these negative thoughts by generating a different view or a "second opinion" about the negative thoughts. To that end, you may want to ask yourself, "Is this thought logical? Is it true?" If not, you can counter it with the truth. If there seem to be common themes to your negative thoughts, you also may want to ask yourself, "Where did I learn this?" You might realize, for example, that you're simply replaying words or scripts from your childhood—perceptions that don't suit you as an adult.

The third, and perhaps most difficult, step in cognitive restructuring is the adoption and implementation of a new frame of mind—substituting positive thoughts for negative ones and sticking with this habit. Much as we're loath to admit it, we're all creatures of habit and we find comfort in familiar ways of being, even if they are maladaptive or stress-inducing. Changing your ways is difficult, and it's easy to revert back to old, unhealthy ways of coping. Once again, what makes a difference is practice—and more practice. If substituting a positive attitude for negative perceptions feels awkward at first, rest assured: As you repeat this conversion, again and again, you'll develop a sense of comfort with the process.

The final step is evaluation: Does this new mindset work? How beneficial is it? The first few attempts might feel artificial or awkward. If, upon further practice, the substitution you've made doesn't sound genuine or right to you and you continue to hear different versions of old negative statements, return to the second step and create a new reappraisal, one that has a greater ring of truth to it.

The techniques used in cognitive restructuring can help train you to monitor the internal monologues that play in your head, whether it's when stress strikes or on a more constant basis. But first, you need to make a record of the thoughts that are flawed by cognitive distortion, those that are bent or twisted out of shape by pessimism, self-criticism, or other forms of negativity. Writing down your self-talk allows you to evaluate your thinking analytically in an effort to clean up errors, distortions, exaggerations, and other faults that perpetuate negative mindsets, bad moods, and the stress response. Then, you can substitute more healthy and positive ways of talking to yourself, ones that will reduce stress and promote your ability to cope. Here's how to internalize this process, step by step:

- **Become aware of your mental chatter.** Over two or three days, pay attention to the kinds of statements you typically make to yourself, or the things you tend to worry or obsess about, and jot these down as accurately as possible. You may want to compare the differences in your internal monologues between the premenstrual and postmenstrual phases of your menstrual cycle. Write down your uncensored thoughts about your situation, mood, or feelings as these negative statements arise.

- **Trace the origins of your negative thoughts.** Ask yourself whether these pessimistic thoughts and worries come from you, from someone else, or from something outside yourself such as a relationship or your work. Do all of your worries stem from one area of your life? In my research, I have found that some women use the heightened sensitivity that occurs premenstrually to their advantage by taking time to think about what's behind some of their negative self-talk, self-criticism, and cognitive distortions. Revealing the source of these negative thoughts can lead to valuable insights about how other people affect your perceptions or how stress overload in certain areas of your life can contribute to a negative mindset. Once you discover where this negativity comes from, it becomes easier to do something about it—when the time is right.

- **Analyze your mental chatter.** Are you friendly toward yourself? Do you compliment yourself? Or are you constantly critical of yourself? Do you make yourself feel guilty? Examine your thoughts for evidence of faulty reasoning, exaggeration, erroneous expectations, or other distortions. Are you labeling yourself unfairly? Are you overemphasizing your shortcomings and mistakes to the exclusion of your strengths and successes? Are you talking yourself into more anxiety or increasing your emotional stress?

- **Reformulate your self-talk in constructive language.** Banish your inner critic and engage in a more helpful dialogue with yourself. Respond to each erroneous thought by writing a more realistic, less polarized, and less exaggerated statement. Let's say you make a huge blunder at work: If you'd normally call yourself an incompetent idiot, you could correct that statement by noting, "I'm not an incompetent idiot. I'm simply a busy woman who made a mistake that can be corrected." These reformulated statements will help to decrease your anxiety and stress response.

Taking time to identify your negative self-talk and use of cognitive distortions can help you on many levels. First, it gives you a time-out, a breather from the multiple, often conflicting, demands on your time. Second, getting rid of negative self-talk will quiet your stress response, resulting in less tension and anxiety. Performing these thought-changing exercises while engaging in deep breathing can add another physiologic dimension to self-calming. And lessening your emotional and physical responses to stressful events in your life can help prevent stress from pumping up the severity of your premenstrual symptoms.

Allison, 27, a graduate student who works part-time as a sales associate, has experienced moderate PMS ever since she began to menstruate at the age of ten. Though physical changes such as cramps, headaches, and acne have been more consistent for her premenstrually, emotional changes such as depression, mood swings, feeling helpless and hopeless, and feeling out of control have been far more debilitating. Twice in her relatively young life, she fell into a clinical depression that she believes stemmed from PMS.

During her participation in the PMS Symptom Management Program at UCSF, she came to realize that some of her cognitive and emotional habits contributed to her mindset's cyclical downward spiral. "Every month, I'd start obsessing about what wasn't going right at school or at work," she explains. "I'd start obsessing about being in a steady relationship and I'd start thinking about breaking up with my boyfriend. Once I started analyzing these recurrent negative thoughts, I realized I had these because I was afraid of getting hurt. I also realized that I'm a perfectionist, and most of the month, I can control my irrational thoughts of perfectionism but not when I am premenstrual."

To overcome these self-defeating habits, "I had to learn how to be more assertive and to be able to ask for what I want without picking a fight," she explains. "I started making lists of my strengths as well as corrective statements when I felt like I wasn't doing anything right. And I had to learn to give myself and other people permission to not be perfect but to do the best job possible and to recognize my achievements even if they're not perfect. Now that I have a better sense of how to take care of my mind and my body, my mood symptoms are much less severe. And my boyfriend and I don't fight premenstrually nearly as much as we used to."

RETRAINING YOUR MIND

Within the arsenal of cognitive restructuring techniques are thought-changing exercises, which can be used to train your mind to rid itself of recurrent negative cogitations or obsessive thoughts. These can also be used with relaxation and meditation techniques if you are having trouble clearing your mind of extraneous clutter. Sometimes, what you need to do is abruptly break the pattern of persistent, negative thoughts and worries. There are two different strategies for doing this: One is called thought-stopping, which basically involves training your mind to halt unwanted thoughts in their tracks. The other is called thought-substituting, in which you rid yourself of negative statements or cognitive distortions by substituting an alternative statement that's positive and accurate.

Thought-stopping entails concentrating on the unwanted thoughts and, after a short time (say, three minutes), suddenly stopping them in midstream and consciously emptying your mind. The command "Stop!" or a loud noise, such as the ringing of a kitchen timer, is generally used to interrupt the unpleasant thoughts. Once you have recognized your stressful thoughts and stopped them, you can use positive self-talk to put yourself in a better state of mind. Here's how to use thought-stopping effectively:

- If you'll be using an alarm, set a kitchen timer or alarm clock for three minutes.

- Sit in a comfortable position and take some slow, deep breaths, relaxing your muscles as you exhale.

- Focus on the worries or negative thoughts that are painful, anxiety-producing, or intrusive.

- Close your eyes and imagine a situation in which the stressful thought is likely to occur; continue to keep the worry in your mind.

- When you hear the alarm ring, shout "Stop!"; you may also want to raise your hand or snap your fingers. Let your mind empty of what you were worrying about; allow only neutral, non-anxious thoughts to remain. Try to keep your mind blank or neutral for at least 30 seconds after the alarm sounds.

- If the negative thoughts or worries return during that time, shout "Stop!" again and repeat the emptying procedure.

Once you have learned this technique, try to take control of the thought-stopping cue without using the timer.

- While focusing on the unwanted thought, shout "Stop!"

- When you succeed in extinguishing the thought this way several times, start interrupting the thought by whispering "Stop!"

- When the whisper becomes sufficient to interrupt the stressful thoughts, simply mouth the word "Stop!" Next, imagine hearing "Stop!" shouted inside your head, then whispered, and so on.

When you can succeed at this stage of the technique, you will be able to stop unwanted thoughts alone or in public, without making a sound or calling attention to yourself. Some women have found that snapping a rubber band around their wrist or pinching themselves when unwanted thoughts occur is a good reminder to put a quick end to this way of thinking.

In addition to being able to stop unwanted thoughts, it's helpful to be able to replace them with healthier ones. To this end, it's important to learn the difference between positive thinking and focusing on the positive. Positive thinking is a matter of expressing hope for the future, perhaps through goal setting, wishful thinking, and dreaming. It can be healthy, but if done to excess, positive thinking can also be a form of denial; after all, you could be denying the reality of today if you focus exclusively on your dreams of a better tomorrow.

Focusing on the positive, by contrast, entails reinterpreting the current situation and appreciating the present moment. You might acknowledge the negative aspects of what's happening but you don't dwell on them; instead, you highlight the positive aspects and build on them. Instead of viewing a rainy day as spoiling your plans for a family hike, you might see it as an opportunity to have lunch together or to go to a matinee. You can also use this concept to reframe negative self-talk in a more positive light. Here's how:

- Sit in a comfortable position and take some slow, deep breaths, relaxing your muscles as you exhale.

- To replace an obsessive or negative thought, conjure up a positive, assertive statement that is appropriate for your situation. If you are feeling overwhelmed by your ever-present list of household chores, instead of telling yourself that you'll never get them done, you might tell yourself, "Most of these responsibilities can be shared or they can wait for another day."

- You may need to develop several alternative statements to say to yourself, since the same response may lose its power with repetition.

Remember that thought-changing takes time. In all likelihood, unwanted thoughts will return and you will have to interrupt them again. The goal should be to stifle the negative thoughts just as they begin to rear their unpleasant heads and to concentrate on something else instead. If you do this, the thoughts will return less and less readily in most cases. And eventually they will cease to be a problem as you retrain your mind with healthier ways of thinking. Practice these strategies throughout the month so that you can consistently reduce your cognitive stress. Once you've made a habit of correcting distorted thoughts, you can use these strategies as you need them.

CHEERING YOURSELF ON

Wouldn't it be great if instead of having a harsh critic living inside your head you had a supportive coach in residence? It's worth trying to make the switch because when you begin to say optimistic, encouraging things to yourself on a regular basis, you'll begin to perceive events differently and you'll be shaping your emotional response to them in a more positive vein.

The idea is to think of kind, supportive things you can say to yourself—whether it's an encouraging mantra or an upbeat affirmation—throughout the day but especially when you feel overwhelmed or undersupported. If you have these words or phrases handy, you can use them as substitutions for negative statements to yourself: If your inner critic often chimes in with "You're not good enough," you might tell yourself "I'm as good as anyone and better than most." It's better still if you can learn to say this regularly before negative self-talk even kicks in. That way, you'll help yourself stay on a more even keel emotionally, and you'll feel better able to cope with whatever circumstances you encounter.

Making this switch can be especially helpful during the premenstrual phase of a woman's cycle, as Janice, 40, an arts consultant, discovered. Here's an example of the sort of monologue that typically played through her head during her premenstrual week:

> *"This has been the worst week of my life. I feel like a complete failure; I just can't seem to do anything right. I know I should be able to do more but every time I try, I just wind up feeling like a loser. I'm beginning to think my PMS will never end. I feel so guilty that my kids see me this way. I know it makes them feel bad and ruins their week, too. I'm helpless in this situation. Every month it's the same thing over and over again; nothing ever changes."*

Upon close scrutiny, it's apparent that this monologue is riddled with cognitive distortions that are likely perpetuating her stress response and negative moods. She is catastrophizing ("This is the worst week of my life"); assigning exaggerated, extreme labels to herself ("failure," "loser," "helpless"); overgeneralizing ("I just can't seem to do anything right"); personalizing the reactions of family members ("it ruins their week, too"); and making erroneous negative predictions ("nothing ever changes"). This adds up to a heavy burden for one woman's shoulders to bear—no wonder she feels so bad premenstrually!

But if she corrected some of these cognitive distortions with a reality check, her self-talk could be used as a potent tool for interrupting the stress cycle. For example, she could rewrite her internal script along these lines:

> *"This week has been more stressful than most. It is also five to seven days before my period starts so I know I may be especially sensitive to stressful events right now. I've also been 'down' on myself this week so*

I've probably exaggerated the importance of relatively minor things that have happened. Of course, my family is affected by my negative mood. I have tried to explain how I am feeling and that it is not their fault. They love me enough to understand; I'm lucky to have them. This difficult week will pass, and hopefully next week will be better for all of us."

In addition to speaking kindly to yourself, it's also a good idea to try to fill up your self-esteem bank so that you can draw upon the balance when you need it most. The truth is, many women focus on their weaknesses rather than their strengths. But you will be doing yourself a big favor if you play up your abilities, accomplishments, and admirable characteristics to the one whose opinion matters most—you. Make a list of these qualities and keep it as a handy reference whenever you feel your self-esteem flagging or you have trouble focusing on your positive attributes. Ask yourself: What do I like about myself? How would other people describe me? What are my special strengths or capabilities? What do I do better than most people? If you really want to improve your self-esteem, the importance of such self-assessment cannot be overemphasized: It is only by cultivating self-awareness that you can consciously and accurately develop a realistic sense of yourself and come to appreciate who you are.

THINKING UP A BETTER REALITY

Not only can cognitive restructuring help bolster your ability to cope with trying situations but it can even help ease stress-related health problems. Research has found, for example, that cognitive restructuring, thought stopping, and thought substitution can decrease the frequency and severity of tension headaches as well as ease the fatigue and functional impairment that are associated with chronic fatigue syndrome. Moreover, a recent study at John Radcliffe Hospital in England found that 12 weekly sessions of cognitive therapy led to a significant decrease in psychological and somatic symptoms, as well as functional impairment, among women with PMS. Meanwhile, in a study at the University of Queensland in Australia, women with premenstrual mood changes who learned how to modify dysfunctional thinking with cognitive restructuring techniques experienced substantial relief from anxiety, depression, and other premenstrual changes.

In my own research, 40 percent of the women with PMS practiced thought-stopping on a daily basis or when they were practicing relaxation techniques. About one-third of the women combined thought-stopping with thought-substitution to control their negative self-talk or toxic thoughts. In the long term, after they had mastered the cognitive and relaxation strategies, more than half of the women used thought-changing strategies "as needed" to control worries or anxiety or to cope with stressful situations.

If you've been allowing negative self-talk to hold center stage in your mind, you have been doing yourself a grave disservice. After all, holding on to negative scripts from the past is as futile as lugging around an oversized suitcase that's packed with outgrown clothes. It's time to give away the garments that no longer fit and treat yourself to a new wardrobe, one that makes you feel good about yourself.

By employing the processes of thought-stopping and thought-substitution, you can become your own best ally by calming yourself down instead of aggravating yourself further. And by reinterpreting events in your life in a more positive, or at least more neutral light, you'll avoid bringing your mood down unnecessarily. Granted, it's easier to refine expectations before an event rather than to try to change your attitude or reframe negative thoughts after the fact. When you find yourself going to a meeting or a social event with preconceived expectations, give them a reality check by questioning their validity and evaluating them to see whether they're appropriate to the situation.

Treat yourself to similarly realistic expectations, too. When you find yourself thinking you "should" do this or that, ask yourself why. What will it accomplish? Who will it help? What will the effect be on you and your loved ones if you do whatever it is you think you should do? And if you don't, who will suffer? In all likelihood, you'll discover that many of the things you told yourself you "should" do can be deferred.

Think of these strategies as a multifaceted approach to stress inoculation, one that occurs from inside your head. Taking these steps will help you avoid feelings of failure and strengthen your sense of self-worth, as well. They'll help you see the bright side of life instead of just the dark side. They'll help you learn how to stop yourself from spiraling downward into a gloomy state of mind. And they'll help you learn how to be good to yourself, which is what you deserve. Best of all, when you treat yourself kindly and gently, life can begin to seem so much more manageable and less threatening, even during the premenstrual phase.

YOUR ASSIGNMENT:

Spend a few minutes thinking about your goals for reducing cognitive stress and which strategies you'd like to start with. To get the ideas percolating, answer the following questions:

- What specific thoughts or negative statements to yourself do you want to change?

- Which of the strategies do you plan to use regularly? Why did you choose those?

- Have you tried cognitive restructuring techniques in the past? If so, are you still using them? If not, why did you stop?

- List as many specific actions and ideas as you can for meeting your goals to change your mindset. (For example, you might choose to follow the cognitive restructuring instructions throughout the month, try the thought-changing exercises to quiet your mind during relaxation sessions, question the "should's" you apply to yourself, and so on.)

- Describe potential obstacles that might thwart your progress (time constraints, negative self-talk, friends who focus on doom and gloom, and the like)—and how you'll deal with them.

- Who will you ask to help or support you in achieving your goals?

8

Managing Your Time Instead of Letting It Manage You

I t's no secret that having a too-full life or a chronically overcrowded schedule can be highly stressful. After all, when the demands on a woman's time exceed the hours in a day, the pressure can feel overwhelming at any time of the month. On a basic level, women often have more to do because they juggle more roles—employee, primary caregiver for children or elderly parents, cook, housekeeper, and so on—than men do. And when a woman is in the premenstrual phase of her cycle, time constraints and an overly hectic schedule can create a climate of sheer chaos, and a woman can easily wind up feeling confused, flustered, and anxious. She might feel as though she's "running around in circles" or "unable to know where to turn or what to do first." Or she may feel like the rabbit in *Alice in Wonderland* who darts about saying, "I'm late! I'm late for a very important date."

While time-management conflicts are often a chronic problem for working women, they become particularly paramount during the premenstrual phase. If a woman isn't feeling her best in the days before the onset of her period, the extra stress that's sparked by poor time management can push her symptoms over the edge—into the debilitating zone. And make no mistake about it: Time-management problems are a very real source of stress, both psychologically and physically. Feeling overwhelmed or overloaded can activate the stress response, as we discussed in Chapter Six. Moreover, the time-crunching juggling act can activate the stress response all day long and into the evening for women. Recent research has found, for example, that working women's stress hormones and blood pressure remain elevated long after the conventional workday is over, unlike men's stress response which typically declines at the end of the workday.

Other studies have revealed that women who have highly demanding jobs, little control in their work, and low social support had the greatest decline in mental and physical functioning over time. These effects may also apply to busy mothers, whether or not they are working, because many of them have too much to do in too little time as they respond to child and family schedules over which they have little control. And even if they had someone to turn to for support, they often can't or don't slow down long enough to think about using the available social support.

The mind-body effects of a rushed lifestyle often become especially apparent during the premenstrual phase of a woman's cycle. The pressure of too much to do in too little time and the physical stress response that's elicited as a result—combined with poor health habits—can exacerbate PMS. Moreover, when your physical and emotional resources are already depleted as you move into the premenstrual phase, you are vulnerable to even the smallest stress response, which can be triggered by time pressures.

Another negative effect of poor time-management is how many women with moderate to severe PMS have very poor health habits. In my research, the majority of these women described themselves as "driven" in terms of their work habits and admitted that they were likely to "keep busy with many activities," especially during the premenstrual period in order to distract themselves from their symptoms. Many were also perpetually "pressed for time" and left time neither for themselves nor for engaging in relaxation activities to cope with their premenstrual symptoms. During the premenstrual phase of their cycles, they reported less satisfaction with themselves and their abilities and a decline in self-esteem. Paradoxically, they began to drive themselves even harder to keep busy, which robbed them further of time for any form of self-care.

THE HAZARDS OF TIME MISMANAGEMENT

The truth is, time management is an essential skill in managing external sources of stress—and in carving out the time you'll need to implement your personalized PMS solution. But numerous habits can sabotage a woman's ability to manage her time effectively. Here are some examples of time-wasting personal habits:

The perfectionist:
The woman who strives for perfection (which is actually unattainable) often gets too caught up in the details of what she's doing and consequently spends too much time on a given project. As a result, she often has little or no free time for health-promoting and stress-reducing activities.

The procrastinator:
This is the woman who adds to her own stress by putting off what she can do today (or right now) for another day. By dragging her feet in completing essential tasks, she makes herself perpetually tardy in fulfilling her responsibilities or obligations. This often has the further effect of diminishing free time.

The time-juggler:
In an attempt to do more in less time, this woman is a master multi-tasker, over-booker, and double-booker who is essentially bargaining for time by trying to do too many things at once. As a result, she is often forced to drop important responsibilities or ends up losing sleep while trying to fulfill all of her obligations.

The can't-say-"no" type:
This woman often derives validation of her self-worth by helping others. She might assume unnecessary responsibilities—such as house-sitting, feeding the neighbor's cat, or driving a friend to the airport—in an effort to gain approval or acceptance. Knowingly or not, those who practice this people-pleasing behavior are often trying to improve their self-esteem but they end up cheating their own needs by doing so much for others.

The poor delegator:

This is the woman who tries to do too many things herself because she hasn't figured out which tasks are appropriate or possible to delegate. Or maybe she feels guilty asking others to help her. Or maybe she is a high achiever and wants to be able to say she's done it all herself. Whatever is at the root of this inability to delegate, it can add up to role overload.

The chronic time underestimator:

This woman perpetually underestimates the amount of time specific activities will require. It could be because she has unrealistic or overly ambitious goals for what she'd like to accomplish in a given day. Or maybe it's because she's easily distracted while working on a particular task so it takes longer than she expects. In any case, she's probably always running behind.

GAUGING THE EXTENT OF THE PROBLEM

In all likelihood, you're no stranger to a time-crunched, self-sacrificing way of living. But are you aware of how big a problem time management is for you? To find out, it helps to give yourself a reality check by figuring out how much time you really spend on different activities in your life. You can use either of the two following methods of time analysis to take an unvarnished look at what you're really doing with your time.

Mapping Your Time.

Keep track of your day or week in 30-minute segments, recording the specific activities and tasks—making a phone call, driving to work, running an errand, preparing meals, watching TV, and so on—that you do in each block of time. Pay attention to how you feel while doing these activities: Do you enjoy doing them? Do you feel anxious or irritable doing them? Are they absolutely necessary for you to do personally? Also, be sure to record what time you go to bed each night and what time you wake up the next day. Note the number of hours that you believe you actually slept: Is this enough for you? Do you feel rested? At the end of the day, divide the day's tasks and activities into categories—work, sleep, driving, cooking, and so on—and add up the time spent in each.

Slicing Your Time Cake:

Draw a circle on a sheet of paper and think of it as a cake that reflects your typical 24-hour day. Start by marking a slice that represents the hours you usually sleep and note the approximate number of hours. Next, mark a slice that reflects the number of hours you typically work outside the home. Chances are, these are the two most substantial slices. Then, draw additional slices to represent how much time you spend traveling to and from work, cooking, cleaning or tidying, taking care of your kids, running errands, exercising, watching TV, talking on the phone, grooming, and so on. Try to be as accurate as possible.

Whether you use the map or the cake method, the next step is to draw up a list of ten activities you truly enjoy—coloring with your kids, going to the movies, reading for pleasure, knitting a sweater, playing the piano, and so on. How many of these are reflected in your time map or cake? The odds are, not many are. The challenge is to look for times when you can fit in some of these by making smart time swaps—perhaps by engaging in one of these pleasurable activities instead of spending two hours watching TV or an hour on the phone at night. This will help restore a sense of balance to your life, as well as helping you to de-stress.

RESTORING A MODICUM OF CONTROL

Let's face it: It's an illusion that you can truly control your life, but you can exert a greater degree of command over the choices you make and the way you use your time. This is especially important during those times of the month when you're not feeling or functioning at your peak. It may be a matter of redefining your roles temporarily, of shifting your priorities, of learning to say "no," and using other essential strategies to make your life easier and less frenetic during the week or so when PMS is likely to strike. But it's also important to get in the habit of doing this all month long to minimize the buildup of stress and tension. It really comes down to taking good emotional care of yourself and allowing yourself to take the time you need to do it.

By the end of the program at UCSF, 80 percent of the women

reported that they used one or more of these time-management strategies on a regular basis. All the women rated learning strategies for managing their time across the menstrual cycle as somewhat to very helpful. Planning and prioritizing the use of time just before the premenstrual phase was rated as the most helpful tactic; however, the strategy of saying "no" in gentle but assertive ways was used the most frequently over the long-term. About one-third of the women found role redefinition—particularly, letting go of certain responsibilities rather than the whole role—to be helpful. Making these changes to their use of time was also linked with improvements in problem-solving abilities and effective communication strategies.

Janice, the 40-year-old arts consultant and mother of two we met in Chapter Seven, typically experienced anxiety, nervousness, sleep problems, fatigue, and irritability, among her constellation of premenstrual symptoms. "My short temper has made me snap at my children when I'm premenstrual, and I usually end up regretting my behavior," she admits. Through the PMS Symptom Management Program, she discovered that planning her weekly schedule in advance helped her avoid overwhelming herself with responsibilities and commitments. It also helped her carve out time for taking walks with her husband, which gave her an opportunity to discuss their mutual schedules and reduce stress together. "At first, I felt guilty taking time for myself because I'd think other people's needs were more important," she recalls. "Making out a weekly schedule helped me see where I was overloading myself."

To lighten her load of responsibilities, she also began talking to her husband about her overburdened "To Do" list and he willingly took on some of those chores. In addition, she reevaluated her roster of work responsibilities and began letting go of a couple of tasks. "Setting limits and learning how to say 'no' was really helpful," she recalls. "After I started changing the way I used my time, I felt much less anxious and tired."

REDEFINING ROLES, CULTIVATING DELEGATING POWERS

Before you can manage your time effectively, it is important to know what you are actually doing along with the amount of time each role takes. Since women typically juggle multiple roles, it's worthwhile to evaluate which roles are "must-do's" or "like-to-do's" and which ones can be effectively delegated to someone else or dropped altogether. On some level, you probably realize that you can't do everything yourself. So why even try when you can delegate some responsibilities to others?

The following exercise will help you examine your various roles or job titles from the perspective of the actual activities or job description each encompasses. Begin by making a list of all the roles that comprise your life—mother, spouse, employee, child-care expert, chauffeur, cook, housecleaner, and so on. Then, using a separate piece of paper for each role, write the role's title at the top of the page and make a list, going down the left side of the page, of all the responsibilities and tasks that make up that role. Be specific: Under "housecleaner," specify that you clean two bathrooms, scour the kitchen, vacuum the entire house, change the sheets, and so on every week rather than simply noting that you clean the house. You can also indicate alongside each of the tasks whether you like to do them (put a + next to those activities), whether you dislike doing them (put a − sign next to these), or whether you feel neutral about these tasks (mark these with a +/− sign).

On the right side of the page, divide the sheet of paper into three columns labeled with the following headings: "Must do myself," "Can delegate with supervision," and "Can delegate completely." Now, go through the list of tasks and responsibilities and ask yourself whether you actually need or want to do each one yourself in order to feel satisfied that it has been accomplished.

The key to mastering the art of delegation is to turn over appropriate tasks—such as those in the third column—to selected people with crystal-clear communication that from now on the task is expected to be entirely their responsibility. This will help clear your mind of the extra stress of keeping tabs on someone else's "To Do" list. If it isn't possible or realistic to completely remove yourself from the picture, try to keep supervision to a minimum. Be clear about your expectations, particularly when it comes to deadlines and desired results; answer questions and check on progress as necessary—but remember to give the person to whom you have delegated the task enough autonomy to do it his or her way, to make his or her own mistakes and to learn by doing so. Try to guard against the urges to criticize, nag, or micromanage. Above all, be sure to thank the person for completing the task; not only is this simple courtesy but it will help reinforce a future willingness to help out.

Granted, it isn't easy to shift your priorities, especially if you've adhered to the same hierarchy for years. It becomes more manageable, however, if you break it down into three primary steps: setting new priorities, scheduling them accordingly, and executing your plan of action. Setting new priorities involves ranking your responsibilities and tasks in their order of importance; you can use the list from your time map or time cake as a starting point. The ABC ranking method involves assigning the letters A, B, or C to various responsibilities: A is for the highest priority activities (those that must be done as soon as possible); B is for second-priority activities (those that must be done soon); and C is for low-priority tasks (things you would like to do but are not essential). Reorder your list of activities in terms of whether they should be on the A list, the B list, or the C list, using the table below.

The ABC Roster

The A List (to be done ASAP)	The B List (must be done soon)	The C List (can wait to be done)
_____	_____	_____
_____	_____	_____
_____	_____	_____
_____	_____	_____

Once you've prioritized your activities, the next challenge is to find the time in which to actually do them. Fortunately, you can use several different techniques to ensure that you have the time to do what needs to get done. The time-blocking method involves dividing your day into five parts: the morning, the noon hour, the afternoon, the dinner hour, and the evening. Write down the significant tasks and assign them a block of time that is most suited to your schedule; be sure to take small breaks during these large blocks of time. If you have a plethora of tasks to do on a particular day, you can use the time-mapping technique to plot out your activities in 30-minute segments throughout the day. Clustering is a variation of the time-blocking method, only in this case responsibilities or tasks are grouped in a sensible way or mapped out by location. This time-saving tactic allows you to complete errands, such as going to the bank and the drycleaner and doing the grocery shopping, that are in close proximity to each other, rather than wasting time running all over town at different times of the day.

RECLAIMING YOUR RIGHTS OF REFUSAL

It's not enough to simply use your time more efficiently. After all, the goal isn't to shoehorn more into an already exhausting schedule. What you'll want to do, instead, is to find sneaky ways to lighten your load of responsibilities. And at some point that's going to require saying "no" to certain requests. Unfortunately, for many women, the phrases that convey refusal, rejection, or other negative responses do not come easily, partly because many of us have been socialized to be sensitive to other people's needs.

It's especially difficult to refuse requests from people you love. And it can be risky to say "no" to superiors at work who can influence the advancement of your job or career. But the risks of not saying "no," at least some of the time, can be even greater because the "yes" habit can set you up for failure of your own goals. When you constantly cater to other people's wants and needs, at the expense of your own, you wind up shortchanging yourself of time to do anything for yourself, whether it's time to relax, engage in a hobby, exercise, practice other forms of self-care, or socialize with your friends. The key to striking some sort of balance between what you do for others and what you do for yourself is to say "no" tactfully, now and then. If you learn to stop saying "no" defensively or tentatively and instead provide respectful but assertive explanations for why you can't comply with a request, you'll feel less guilt and anxiety about your decision and you'll increase the quality of your communication skills. For example, if a colleague asks you to read her report in the midst of a particularly stressful day, you could say, "I'd love to be able to help you out, but I won't be able to today." If your husband requests that you pick out a tie for him just as you were trying to get out the door, you could say, "No, I'm sorry but I just don't have time to." And if your four-year-old begs you to play with him while you are trying to get dinner on the table, you might say, "Honey, I can't right now but I'd love to after dinner." Just make sure that your body language doesn't undermine your message: You'll need to use direct eye contact, erect posture, a pleasant expression of firmness on your face, and so on to reinforce your message.

The next step is to apply these techniques to real situations where you might want to say "no." When someone makes a request of you, don't answer automatically. Build in a pause and listen to your inner voice: Does the request make you feel resentful? Anxious? Fearful? If so, think about why that is the case. If you need time to figure out why you don't want to do something, stall by telling the person that you will get back to her soon. If the request will interfere with the time you'd like to devote to self-care or your PMS plan—and it's not essential for you to do—these are reasons enough to say "no." After all, these activities deserve to rise to a prominent position on your priority list.

PUTTING THESE STRATEGIES INTO PRACTICE

As the saying goes, time waits for no one so it's up to you to start reclaiming control over how you spend your time. As we've suggested, managing your time—whether this involves setting priorities, being realistic about how long activities will take, keeping a calendar or "To Do" list, saying "no" after considering the consequences, or building in time to deal with unexpected crises—will help alleviate stress, particularly during the premenstrual phase.

When you have a clear idea of where to focus your efforts, you'll want to start practicing your time-management skills on a regular basis. Think of this as a way to work and live smarter, rather than harder. Use whatever tools—clocks, calendars, day planners, priority lists, and "To Do" lists—you need to stay organized and focused on your top priorities. Assign deadlines to specific tasks and activities to help yourself stay on schedule. Share responsibilities for household chores and errands with your spouse, whenever possible, and delegate tasks that aren't essential for you to do. Practice saying "no" to requests and invitations you can't or don't want to fulfill. And try to build in some flexibility for emergencies, pleasant surprises, unexpected visitors, a child's illness, and so on so that your schedule isn't always packed around the clock.

Employing these strategies on a regular basis can help you avoid feeling perpetually pressed for time and stressed out. But you may want to crank up your diligence with these techniques during the premenstrual phase of your cycle, particularly if you often feel less efficient or competent on those days. Managing your days effectively can also help you carve out precious time—ideally, a minimum of 30 minutes a day—to tend to your own needs and to implement your PMS plan. There's no question that that is time well spent.

YOUR ASSIGNMENT:

Spend a few minutes thinking about the goals you'd like to set for managing your time more effectively. This will help you make practical choices and anticipate what might be involved. To get the ideas flowing, answer the following questions:

☐ What specific changes are you willing to make to manage your time or your "To Do" list?

☐ Which aspects of time management have you struggled with in the past—and how did you handle them?

☐ List as many concrete actions and ideas as you can for meeting your time-management goals.

☐ Now think about potential obstacles that might stand in your way (last-minute crises, unsupportive people, your inner naysayer, not allocating enough time to activities, and the like)—and how you'll deal with them.

☐ Who will you ask to help or support you in achieving your goals?

9

The Relationship Dance of PMS

"*I don't mean for it to happen but my husband becomes my emotional punching bag when I have PMS. I guess I feel like he can take my lashing out at him better than my kids can. But I know I'm driving him away when I scream at him. If only he'd help me out without me having to ask or if he'd just ask me instead of waiting for me to tell him what to do, this wouldn't be an issue.*"

There's no question that some women feel as though they're on an emotional high wire during the premenstrual phase of their cycles. Everyday annoyances and hassles can seem magnified, sometimes exponentially, and it can be especially hard to cope with aggravation and stress when you're already feeling out of sorts physically and emotionally. Of course, it's hardly surprising that PMS can create problems in your relationships at home or at work. But when interpersonal conflicts arise, these sources of stress can increase the severity of your premenstrual symptoms.

Part of the problem may be that you're too reactive to what's going on around you and that you've temporarily become an emotional loose cannon. As a result of this unusually short fuse, you may be reacting more strongly to aggravating factors, and this, in turn, gets you more riled up. Meanwhile, you might become more short-tempered or impatient than usual with those around you, which can elicit emotional reactions from them that perpetuate your tense feelings. Before you know it you're engaged in the edgy dance of PMS. By now, you've undoubtedly realized that PMS doesn't affect you exclusively. In fact, in a study at the University of Washington in Seattle, researchers found that 75 percent of men reported that their lives were moderately to greatly disrupted by their partners' PMS.

▪ *Just For Him* ▪

Is your partner in the dark about what it feels like to have PMS? If so, it's time to have a chat about your physical, emotional, and cognitive symptoms as well as how he can help. Tell him that it's hard for you to function as well as usual. Ask him how your PMS affects him. Take deep breaths if you feel anxious or defensive about what he has to say. If you have a hard time getting the conversation started, ask him to read this section which addresses questions frequently asked by men, then reconvene for a tête-à-tête.

- *How does PMS affect a man's life?*

If you have been living with a woman who experiences PMS, you may feel as though you have a period, too. But just because you've lived through her cyclical ups and downs, don't assume that you know how it feels. To find out, ask her: What is PMS like for you? What does it feel like? Also, consider how her cyclical changes affect you: Do you feel tense when you know her premenstrual days are approaching? Do you find yourself becoming more reactive than usual to things she says or does? If so, you may want to engage in activities such as exercise that reduce your own stress response.

- *Is PMS contagious?*

Some men describe feeling as though they have PMS, too, or the women in their lives notice their men have cyclical reactions such as feeling edgy or tense as the premenstrual phase approaches. Intimate relationships are dynamic—one person's behavior triggers a reaction in the other and vice versa. If this happens over and over again, these responses can become automatic. The menstrual cycle—like all strong, predictable biological rhythms—has a stabilizing effect on our own bodies and behavior as well as the bodies and behavior of our loved ones through pheromones, hormones that are transmitted through the sense of smell. When the rhythm is peaceful and regular, a woman's partner may not even notice his reactions. But when storm clouds move in, as they do with PMS, her partner may overreact to her behavior or experience a heightened stress response to her ups and downs.

■ *Are your needs getting short shrift during the premenstrual phase?*

Some men feel hurt by their partners' angry outbursts or confused by the mixed messages that are often sent during this phase of the menstrual cycle. It is important to communicate these feelings to her in ways that she can hear (see some of the constructive communication strategies described in this chapter). You will be able to be more supportive of her if you can acknowledge or resolve your own resentments.

■ *How can you help her?*

Start by working with her on her personalized PMS plan—without trying to take over and fix what she's going through. Ask questions such as "What can I do to be helpful?" and "How can we act as a team in working on your PMS plan?" Let her take the lead but think about what you can do—make dinner, play with the kids, assume responsibilities for certain household chores—so that she'll have the time she needs to implement her chosen strategies. You might also suggest keeping a calendar to alert both of you to when her premenstrual phase is likely to begin.

■ *How can you help yourself?*

When emotions reach the boiling point or premenstrual life feels especially stressful, sometimes the best thing to do is take a "time-out"—not a passive withdrawal or a hostile escape but some negotiated time to cool down or be alone. Sometimes men feel helpless in the face of rapid mood swings and tearfulness, but silently withdrawing isn't the answer. That's likely to feel like abandonment to her. Getting angry doesn't help, either. Anger begets anger: It's like the dance of PMS. (If you respond with anger rather than with offers of support, you might want to read the section on anger management in Chapter Ten.) If you tend to respond in these ways, you're hardly alone: In one study, 75 percent of men coped with PMS by expressing anger, withdrawing, or ignoring the situation.

Instead, it's better to take some deep breaths, count to five in your head, and suggest that you take a break from the topic of discussion. The two of you can negotiate a mutually agreeable time to resume your conversation, without the hostile or argumentative salvos. When possible, it is often helpful to reschedule heated discussions for a time in the post-menstrual phase—meaning, after her period has ended.

The truth is, no matter how many stress-reduction strategies you try, there are many harsh realities in the world that cannot be eliminated by a change in attitude or outlook. But if you can identify potential minefields in your relationships that tend to trip you up most consistently, and you can learn to defuse them in some way, you'll be paving a smoother path for yourself. The first step is to pinpoint sources of stress in your relationships with family, friends, and coworkers, and to determine when the problem is yours and when the problem belongs to someone else. If it's yours, you can try to modify it in a favorable way. If it's the other person's and you don't want it to become your problem, you can find ways to shield yourself from it, thereby protecting yourself from further anxiety, worry, or mood swings. Not only is this valuable for your general sense of well-being, but it's an important component of your personal PMS plan, too.

In my own research, prior to treatment, 80 percent of the women with PMS rated their stress as moderately high to very high. Overall, they rated their work as very stressful, their relationships and family life as moderately stressful, and their physical health and parenting roles as not very stressful. As we mentioned in Chapter Six, women with more severe PMS were more likely to have a heightened reaction to stress than women with less severe PMS. We also found that while some women had "stress buffers" such as good relationships with children, spouses, or friends, or positive self-esteem or feelings of general well-being, these diminished during the premenstrual phase: In particular, feelings of well-being and self-esteem dropped markedly—by up to 30 percent—during the week before the women's periods arrived. Many women reported that this change was related to the impact of PMS on their relationships, both at work and at home. They also reported that they felt particularly bad about their ability to communicate and cope with relationship stress. Not surprisingly, their stress levels, particularly in relation to work and relationships, tended to rise during the premenstrual phase.

CYCLES OF GRIPING AMONG SPOUSES

What I've found, in my research, is that both men and women often claim that the other uses PMS as an excuse for not having sex, for not doing his or her share of domestic chores, or for myriad problems in their relationship. Time and again, women and their spouses or partners would tell us about the problems that PMS caused in their relationship and how destructive their communication patterns would become.

> *"He says, 'Your period is about to start; you're whining' . . . I think he just uses PMS as an excuse to not pay attention to me."*
>
> *"My breasts get tender for about two weeks and I don't want my husband to touch me. He thinks I'm just making excuses; he doesn't understand. Then he gets mad and when I want to have sex, after I'm feeling better, he just turns away. Thanks to PMS, sex has become a power struggle between us."*

Over time, couples typically become more and more defensive with their partners, in an effort to protect themselves against verbal attacks. They stop listening to each other, believing that they know what the other really means or thinking they know what the other will say in response. As a result, they jump to conclusions before the other has a chance to finish a sentence. For some women, unexpressed resentments build to a crescendo and get released in a torrent of rage, or their inability to communicate effectively or negotiate with their partners leads to a growing mountain of resentments. Unresolved conflicts pile up for both partners, resulting in a suppression of love and respect for the other.

Given this communication breakdown, it's no wonder many women describe their monthly "PMS divorce" as a time when they feel hopeless about their relationships or marriages, when they think all their loving feelings have been permanently extinguished. Then, they get their periods, and suddenly all is forgotten or forgiven. These feelings dissipate. Hope returns. Once again, they're a "we" and happy about it. (Men may take a little longer to return to this state: Research at the University of Washington in Seattle found that men's marital dissatisfaction often continues through the woman's period and into the post-menstrual phase. In other words, men can experience an emotional hangover that can last for weeks.)

Those loving feelings aren't the only aspects of a romantic relationship that can ebb and flow. For many women, sexual desire, as well as the need for closeness and intimacy, also go through monthly cycles. As Theresa L. Crenshaw, M.D., points out in her book *The Alchemy of Love and Lust,* many women experience a mild sexual peak—especially in desire—at midcycle but an even stronger one premenstrually. "During this time, genital sensations revive, and orgasm is easier to achieve," she notes. "Sexual sensitivity simmers."

In my own research, some women have described this sensation as feeling "sexually charged." Yet because they also feel irritable, tense, anxious, and overwhelmed, many women lash out at their partners in anger or grapple with resentments that may have been building during this time. As a result, there's a paradoxical response during the premenstrual phase: A woman may want to have sex but she may not want to talk to her partner in order to control her hostile feelings. Her partner may feel confused by the sexual come-on and the emotional distance. If her partner withdraws from sexual intimacy, the premenstrual woman may experience sexual frustration, which may increase her turmoil symptoms.

"The effects of PMS have been very bad on my relationships," confesses Anne, 37, a financial analyst who lives with her boyfriend. "I have been with many wonderful men but PMS eventually wears them out. I don't like being out of control emotionally; I don't like feeling dependent. I don't like that I nag my partner, that I'm not loving and supportive. I end up sending mixed messages—first, I am clingy and needy when I'm premenstrual but then when my partner tries to respond, I push him away or get angry that he's not doing this or that in the right way. It's no wonder they give up and go away after a while. I guess I would, too."

Meanwhile, those women who become hypersensitive to touch during the premenstrual phase may shy away from sexual intimacy because their partners don't touch them in a way that feels good. If these women don't find a way to communicate to their partners what feels good, this response can also cause hurt feelings and withdrawal. Some women use masturbation as a way to deal with their need for sexual release; others find that gentle massage by their partners helps to calm the hypersensitive sensations. The latter option can be appealing to those women who really crave closeness and cuddling, rather than sexual intimacy, during the premenstrual phase.

PMS ON THE HOME FRONT

Of course, romantic relationships are not the only ones that get buffeted by PMS. As you've undoubtedly recognized, PMS affects the whole family. And many women describe their guilt and anguish about the effects of PMS on their children, in particular. As Jennifer, 38, a stay-at-home mother, confesses, "When I have PMS, I want to be left alone and that scares my five-year-old son so he gets even more clingy with me. Then, I become more forceful and make him stay in his room so that I can be alone. I pray that my husband will come home early so he can take over for me. But when he does come home, my son runs to him for protection from me. And I feel like an ogre. My husband worries that I might be acting abusively toward our son, and then we end up fighting, too."

Other women fear that PMS makes them act inconsistently as parents. Sometimes, they might be kind and permissive; other times, they may be strict and hotheaded—and these fluctuations in their behavior often coincide with changes in their menstrual phase but not always in a predictable way. Some of the women in my research, for example, confessed to bribing their kids with candy or junk food or extra TV-watching privileges, just so they could carve out some time for themselves. Not surprisingly, many women worry about the toll this inconsistency will take on their children over the long run. As one woman explains, "When my PMS is bad, I act impulsively and make premature decisions or impose unnecessary punishments with my kids. I don't think rationally about what the consequences are so I'll make snap decisions about what they can and can't do. And it just makes things worse. They get all worked up and I feel bad because I don't feel like a very good parent."

PMS ON THE WORK FRONT

Another factor that can increase PMS severity is work stress. In one study, about 15 percent of the women reported that relationship problems at work—such as increased conflicts, criticism, complaints, and rejection—increased the severity of their PMS. These findings were confirmed in my own research. It's not just the communication problems with individual coworkers that are stressful to women with PMS. Often, the overall work environment can place an added strain on women during the premenstrual phase. Women with PMS often report being more sensitive to noise, temperature changes, odors, and nonverbal tension among coworkers or work groups. Conflicting demands from various managers or supervisors or a lack of control over how the work is performed can also be especially tough to take premenstrually. Not surprisingly, women often report increased stress due to excessive workloads or insufficient time to complete their work during this already difficult time in their menstrual cycles.

Another burden and added source of stress for women with PMS is the feeling that they must conceal their premenstrual symptoms from their coworkers or supervisors. Sometimes it is safe to confide in a coworker about your PMS but each work relationship and situation is different because there is the concern that you might be discounted or perceived negatively if others know you have PMS. This was certainly true for Margaret, 35, a research scientist who worked in a laboratory where she was the only woman. "At work, I feel the most stress," she says. "On some premenstrual days, the pressure seems to build and I feel like my head is going to explode. I feel desperate but I hold it all in and withdraw from my colleagues. It's not that the guys aren't great to work with; it's just such a fast-paced environment and I get the feeling that if I don't keep up then I won't be one of the guys. Sometimes I see them looking at me, wondering what's going on but I don't talk about it. I also hear them talking about their own wives and girlfriends, saying things like, 'I have to be careful—she's on the rag' or 'She's so irrational—it must be PMS.' I don't want them to know I have PMS because I don't want to be labeled by them."

In my early studies of women with PMS, we found that many women were not aware of how work stress affected the severity of their symptoms. While a number of women rated their work as highly stressful, for example, they had difficulty specifying the nature of the stress. Upon further questioning, it became apparent that conflicts with coworkers or supervisors were the most common source of stress, but it wasn't until we actually observed their work settings that we began to see a pattern of physical, psychological, and social sources of stress in the work environment.

A case in point: Lucy, 28, a legal secretary at a large law firm, attributed her job stress to her long commute. Yet, when we asked to meet her at her work setting at a prearranged time, we immediately observed numerous physical and environmental sources of stress, including a negative tone in the office. When we first entered, we encountered a receptionist who was abrupt, curt, and unfriendly in her demeanor. People were rushing down the hall, yelling for other people to assist them immediately; the atmosphere was charged with pressure. Lucy worked in a small cubicle that was surrounded by 20 similar cubicles, all of which were occupied. As a result, she had little sound privacy and could easily hear conversations from other cubicles. During the average day, she reported being distracted by other cubicle conversations or interrupted by phone calls about every five minutes.

In this particular study, we measured the stress levels and stress hormones of female employees. Although many women reported high levels of work-related stress, only those women who experienced a high degree of physical and/or psychosocial stress in their work environment—women like Lucy—exhibited very high levels of stress hormones. Among the women who were able to modify their work environment to reduce stress, we found a corresponding reduction in their physiologic stress response, as measured by stress hormones. But this did not happen for the women who did not or could not change their stressful work situations. Lucy, for example, had tried to make changes in her work setting—by talking to the office manager about helping coworkers, decreasing the ambient noise, initiating flexible work hours, and so on—but neither her stress level nor her hormonal response declined until she quit her job.

Putting Together Your Own Support Group

Study after study has found that social support can buffer the effects of stress, chronic illness, personal loss, and change. It can also boost your self-esteem and feelings of well-being and help you implement health-promoting goals. So why wouldn't it help with PMS? The truth is, it can. But the challenge is to get the right kind of support.

In my research at UCSF, women were encouraged to incorporate peer support into their personal PMS plans. Surprisingly enough, those with a long history of PMS reported a lack of trust in other women with similarly severe symptoms. Their feeling was "Why should I trust someone who is as miserable as I am and for as long?" Once women had begun to individualize their PMS management regimens, however, they used the peer support group to help them fine-tune their programs and reinforce the success of their treatments. Among the elements that made peer support effective were reassurance of self-worth, encouragement, respect, positive reinforcement in making difficult behavioral changes, and information and treatment recommendations. Most women perceived the group experience as helpful, especially because it afforded them an opportunity to hear how others modified their treatment strategies. But some women thought they could reap similar benefits from a supportive group of friends.

Whether you form a PMS support group or identify a friend or two to help you implement your PMS plan, most women find that it's helpful to have supportive relationships with other women who experience PMS. That way, you can commiserate, empathize, and help each other with suggestions on how to ease your symptoms. But the relationship must be supportive. Though you may not be able to stay away from friends or family members who are stress inoculators, you can try to minimize your contact with them, especially during your premenstrual days. Then, when you feel better after the arrival of your period, you can try to make up for lost time.

EVERYDAY TALK THERAPY FOR PMS

Many women find it harder to communicate during their premenstrual days than at other times of the month. This may be because effective, respectful, or loving communication doesn't come naturally when you're feeling sad, angry, or cranky. When you're feeling revved up or frazzled, you may not consider how to choose your words carefully. Or you may not listen fully to other people's responses. Once you develop these communication habits, it will take a concentrated effort on your part to undo them.

To be an effective communicator, you must not only express thoughts and feelings in understandable words and actions but listen, clarify, and process information as it is intended. Interpersonal communication needs to be clear and direct—you must say what you mean and mean what you say. Most of us have never been trained to be effective communicators, and we may think that talking to people requires common sense and nothing more. But common sense can be muffled or distorted by emotions like anxiety, depression, irritability, or anger—emotions that are activated during stress and PMS and can impair a woman's ability to gather, process, and exchange information. This impairment leads to miscommunication and the stress that miscommunication engenders.

"To me, it's like truth serum—I just can't hide my emotions when I'm premenstrual," confesses Lisa, 29, a marketing executive. "People misunderstand me or they feel hurt by what I say. Then I feel bad about not being more tactful. I should probably wait until I feel better to say something."

Indeed, sometimes it's better to write down how you're feeling in a journal than to simply speak out impulsively. You can always decide to broach the subject at a later date—in a more diplomatic fashion. This stalling tactic can help you avoid damaging your relationships. After all, when miscommunication occurs frequently, people have a tendency to withdraw from each other and relationships deteriorate. Self-esteem can also take a downturn in the process. On the other hand, learning to communicate calmly and effectively has been found to help people deal with depression, anger, resentment, and anxiety that may stem from problems in relationships with family members, colleagues, friends, or other people. The key is to be able to express the essence of your PMS experience in terms of what you want and expect from other family members. When women learn to state exactly what they feel and need, there is often a collective sigh of relief from family members. Why? Because they no longer have to try to read your mind or guess what you want.

In talking to your family about what it feels like to have PMS, describe your feelings as clearly as possible. You might tell them that sometimes you feel like a prisoner in your own body, that you dislike how you act toward yourself and others, and that you become frustrated and powerless as you try to make changes that don't seem to work. Remember that your family would rather empathize with you than be criticized by you. Reassure your children that they are not the source of your problems. They may be young but don't underestimate their ability to understand or empathize. Try to be as clear as possible without giving too much information. You might say, "I'm dealing with PMS, which is a problem that affects my body and my mood, too. Sometimes it makes me feel bad all over. I know that I'm not easy to live with and that this can be a tough time for you, too. I really appreciate your support and patience." Acknowledging the problem shows your children that you care about their feelings. It will also give them some insight into how they can best interact with you. You might even ask your kids for their opinions and suggestions about how you can help each other through this difficult time.

WHAT'S YOUR COMMUNICATION STYLE?

Before you can revamp or fine-tune your communication skills, you'll need to figure out how you—and those who are closest to you—tend to communicate. Each of us has her own distinct style of communication that has been influenced by geography, experience, family values, as well as formal and informal education. When communication styles are markedly different or provoke emotional responses in the listener, conflicts and miscommunication develop, resulting in an activation of the stress response and negative emotions. What's more, over time, many people develop bad habits in the way they use language or mannerisms that distract from the message, without even being aware that they're setting up barriers to respectful, clear communication. When attempting to communicate while under stress or while experiencing PMS, a person's communication style can become exaggerated, which often widens the chasm of misunderstanding.

In her book *That's Not What I Meant!*, linguistics expert Deborah Tannen suggests that most Americans tend to be indirect rather than direct in the way we communicate, whether it's out of politeness, fear, or manipulation. In her research, she has found that indirect communication, both verbal and nonverbal, leads to increased stress and potential conflicts among people that perpetuate the use of indirect communication.

While there are many different communication styles, they can be classified into four primary categories—aggressive, passive, passive-aggressive, and direct:

The aggressive style:
Whether it's through sparring, accusing, threatening, blaming, labeling, interrupting, or verbally stepping on people, the aggressive com-

municator is able to control professional or social situations and feels a sense of reward in getting what she wants. This feeling of gratification encourages future attempts to dominate, namely by talking too much or interrupting others. An aggressive communicator might say to her partner, "Am I your maid or what? I'm pissed off because you never help with the dishes. You don't care what happens around here!" Not surprisingly, this sort of behavior is often met with defensive, intimidated, or hostile responses. Over time, the aggressive communicator may alienate herself from others.

The passive style:

With this style, a person usually withholds her thoughts, desires, feelings, and ideas in an effort to avoid confrontation, tension, and conflict. Sometimes the nonassertive person is afraid to admit even to herself how intensely she feels about something so she may use hedge phrases, a soft or hesitant voice, an averted gaze, or timid body language. A passive communicator might ask her spouse, "I'm sorry to bother you but would you mind terribly wiping the dishes?" Because this style naturally puts someone else in charge of decision-making, the passive communicator may feel anxious about how things will turn out or disappointed or angry with herself for not trying to take more control.

The passive-aggressive style:

We all know it when we see it because it's something we've all encountered. The woman with this style exhibits a combination of the worst of the aggressive and passive styles. The passive-aggressive communicator might use sarcasm or humor as a weapon then become passive or withholding in the face of conflict. She might accuse, label, or manipulate others then, when confronted with her behavior, claim to be seriously misunderstood. In other words, she fluctuates widely in her approach with the result being that you're never sure what to expect from her.

The direct style:

A more honest and straightforward approach is the direct communication style, which is sometimes referred to as assertive communication. Someone who communicates directly and assertively stands up for herself, expresses her true feelings, and doesn't let others take advantage of her. At the same time, she is considerate of other people's feelings and is willing to listen to other people's ideas without worrying about being manipulated or intimidated. Her personal preferences are stated in clear, non-antagonistic terms, and with sufficient consistency that others know what to expect. This style of communication relies heavily on statements that begin with "I": "Honey, I would like you to dry the dishes as I wash them."

REVAMPING YOUR INTERPERSONAL STYLE

One of the most important things to learn about effective, assertive communication is that you need to have a goal. In other words, you need to be clear about what you need or want from an encounter—as well as what you do not want to happen. To make sure you don't overlook any of the important aspects of direct communication, it helps to break the process down to its essential parts, using what we call the "CANDOR" technique. CANDOR is actually an acronym that serves as a mnemonic device to help you remember the steps that are vital for effective communication.

C   **Consider** what you want, need, and feel about the situation, as well as how the other person is likely to feel about it.

A   **Arrange** a convenient time and place to discuss the issue with the other party.

N   **Name** the problem then describe what happened, when and where it happened.

D   **Describe** your feelings calmly and directly, using "I" statements like "I feel hurt."

O   **Outline** your request for change with a simple sentence or two.

R   **Reinforce** the chances of getting what you want by describing a positive consequence of cooperating.

Here's an example of how Sarah, 42, a real estate agent, used the "CANDOR" technique to gain her spouse's help with implementing her PMS plan:

Consider: "I need to schedule some time for myself, and it's my responsibility to make sure that Jim understands my need to launch my PMS plan."

Arrange: "I'll ask him if he's willing to discuss this when he gets home tonight. If he isn't, we'll set a time and place to talk about it in the next day or two."

Name: "I've been interrupted during my relaxation practice more than once in the last week. Jim says he'll play with the kids but then they wander up to my room or Jim yells through the door, asking me where something is."

Describe: "I feel angry, frustrated, and hurt when my time alone is impinged upon. This also makes it harder for me to continue practicing."

Outline: "I would like not to be interrupted while I practice my relaxation exercises for 30 minutes, three days a week—unless it's a dire emergency."

Reinforce: "If I'm not interrupted, I'll be more successful with my PMS plan and I'll feel better more quickly. Also, I am willing to give Jim the same kind of time to himself, if he needs it."

As you can see, Sarah's script is specific and detailed. Her statement of the problem is clear and to the point, without blaming anyone or apologizing for what she's asking for. She is expressing her feelings using "I" statements and she is linking them to specific events or behaviors, without judging anyone. In other words, she isn't blaming Jim for letting her down; she is simply stating unequivocally what she needs from him. Using these tactics, she's more likely to get it.

The same communication principles apply to work relationships, except that you may want to be circumspect about describing your PMS experience—or asking for help with it. Instead of divulging your monthly secret, you may want to focus on developing communication skills that will reduce relationship stress and help you to become more efficient and competent in your work environment. This can help ease your premenstrual symptoms indirectly as well as improving the quality of your work life.

■ *Cultivating a Can-Do Spirit* ■

The philosophy behind the "CANDOR" technique can also be applied to solving problems that stem from sources of stress that lie outside your relationships. If you remove the R at the end of candor, you're left with CAN DO. You can use the same steps from the communication-improving technique to bolster your ability to handle various stressful challenges, whether it's asking your boss for a raise, coping with a financial crisis, or dealing with a child's behavior problems at school. Here's an example of how you could put it into action:

C　**Consider** what you want, need, and feel about the problem at hand, then examine the other side of the issue.

A　**Arrange** a convenient time and place to discuss the issue with others who are involved.

N　**Name** the nature of the problem as well as when, where, and how long it's been going on.

D　**Describe** your feelings calmly and directly, using "I" statements like "I feel concerned because . . ."

O　**Outline** what you would like to happen with a simple sentence or two.

Taking this approach to daunting challenges can help increase your sense of control over the matter by putting you in problem-solving mode. Rather than getting stuck on the emotional side of the issue, you will be looking at possibilities for change. You will be addressing the problem directly, instead of avoiding or denying it. And you will be taking charge of doing something about it, which always feels empowering.

You can use the CANDOR technique as a tool to practice communicating more effectively. Think about a recent encounter that proved to be problematic and write out a script, using the CANDOR steps, for how you could have handled it more constructively. If you learn to apply these principles to your personal history and you practice restyling your communication skills along these lines, eventually you'll be able to do this with new situations as they arise.

Of course, it's important to make sure your body language is supporting what you're saying. Although nonverbal messages—forms of touch, physical gestures, facial expressions, voice pitch or volume, and the use of personal space—can support or reinforce verbal messages, they can also contradict the spoken words, resulting in confusing or mixed messages. Research has suggested that 70 percent of communication is transmitted through nonverbal cues so it's important to make sure that your body language is in tune with the message you're trying to send. Folding your arms across your chest, for example, or crossing your legs away from a speaker may or may not indicate boredom, defensiveness, or aggression but you should be aware that someone could read these cues that way. Realizing that communication involves both verbal and nonverbal messages, you can use the following five guidelines about nonverbal communication to make your overall communication style as effective as possible:

1. Maintain direct eye contact but don't stare.

2. Maintain erect body posture (head tall, shoulders back, and so on).

3. Speak clearly, audibly, and firmly.

4. Don't whine or have an apologetic tone to your voice.

5. Use gestures and facial expressions to emphasize your points.

Practicing these in front of a mirror can help you observe how other people may perceive your body language.

Overcoming Resistance From Others

By following the recommended steps for improving communication, you will likely gain a sense of confidence and control in dealing with other people. But the element of control can be somewhat illusory because things won't always go according to your plan. You may, in fact, encounter resistance from others when you change your behavior, even if the change is for the better.

You may find that some people will ignore your direct requests. Others may try to bully you into adopting their point of view. Still others may simply deny the validity of what you're telling them. Fortunately, there's something you can do ahead of time to prepare for these possibilities—arm yourself with clever strategies to circumvent these tactics. Here's a grab bag of communicative tricks to help you do just that:

Sound like a broken record: If someone doesn't appear to be listening to you or attempts to delay or deny your request, calmly repeating your point without getting sidetracked or emotional can be quite effective. Your lines might go something like this: "I'd really like to be able to talk about this . . . Yes, I know you're busy, but we really need to find some time to talk about this . . . It sounds like you don't want to talk about this but this is important to me . . . I really need your help so I'd like to talk to you about this . . ." What you want to do is keep an even tone to your voice, maintain direct eye contact, and continue repeating your request until it is heard.

Defuse intense feelings: When your own emotions or someone else's appear to be spiraling out of control, this technique serves as a much-needed "time-out" that defers the discussion until you've both had a chance to calm down. To achieve this, you might say, "I can see that you're pretty upset right now. Why don't we discuss this later this afternoon?"

Put off the discussion respectfully: When a challenging statement puts you at a loss for words, use this strategy to put off a response until you feel calmer and better able to deal with the situation constructively. You might say, "Hmm. That's a very interesting point . . . I'll have to mull that over for a little while . . . Let's talk about this again later." This technique may be especially helpful when you're afraid that you'll burst into tears and you need to take a break.

Ask for more information: When you feel as though you are under attack and you don't understand why, you can use this strategy to elicit more information or to clarify the situation. What you want to do is essentially prompt criticism—by saying something like "I understand that you don't like the way I acted at the meeting last night. What is it about my behavior that bothered you?"—so that you can gather the information you need to respond effectively. This is a good strategy to use when you feel emotionally stable and ready to hear what the other person has to say.

A SCRIPT FOR CHANGE

Like most skills in life, learning to communicate more effectively takes time and practice. But the effort is worth it when you consider the potential payoff. By the end of the study at UCSF, two-thirds of the participants found that learning effective communication and problem-solving strategies was helpful. After initiating their personal PMS plans, 50 percent of the women practiced using assertive communication in the short-term and 66 percent continued using effective communication strategies over the long-term. Through improved communication, women reported feeling better about themselves and their relationships.

Of course, effective communication requires good listening and responding skills, too. Listening is different than hearing; it requires attending to what the other person is saying, processing it, and understanding it. The secret to truly listening is to clear your mind of all thoughts and to pay attention to what the speaker is really saying. To help yourself process the information, you can paraphrase or summarize what the person is saying or ask questions to enhance the clarity of what you're hearing. This will ensure that the messages are flowing freely in both directions.

<u>YOUR ASSIGNMENT:</u>

Take some time to consider your goals for reducing stress in your relationships and think about which strategies you'd like to start with. To get the creative juices flowing, answer the following questions:

☐ What specific communication problems do you want to change? Who are they related to—your intimate partner, child, boss, coworker, other family members?

☐ Which ineffective communication styles do you practice and want to change?

☐ Have you tried doing this in the past? If so, what prevented you from succeeding?

☐ List as many specific actions and ideas as you can for meeting your goals to improve your communication skills.

☐ Describe potential obstacles that might thwart your progress (time constraints, negative self-talk, temperamental people in your life, and the like)—and how you'll deal with them.

☐ Who will you ask to help or support you in achieving your goals?

10

Putting the Pieces Together

By now, you've read about the various ways in which modifying your lifestyle and your environment can help with PMS. You've discovered the secrets to sound nutrition and exercise that will help eliminate some of the premenstrual symptoms that may crop up month after month. You've learned about the importance of taking time to de-stress regularly. You've seen how miscommunication can flare up during the premenstrual phase and aggravate a woman's already irksome symptoms. And you've learned how other women have used various PMS management strategies in their own lives. Now it's time to put all this newfound wisdom to good use in your life by figuring out how to structure your own PMS solution. This is the part where it's up to you to set personal goals for how you want to feel and function and to choose your strategies accordingly. Just remember to try to have realistic expectations and remind yourself that perfection is not the goal here.

If the prospect of putting together a personalized PMS plan seems overwhelming at this point, don't worry: We'll show you how to do it step by step and week by week. If you haven't yet tracked your symptom severity for one menstrual cycle, go back to Chapter Three and follow the instructions for tracking your symptoms, identifying your most bothersome or severe forms of discomfort, and determining your premenstrual mood pattern. Without this vital information, you cannot create a custom-tailored solution to your premenstrual woes.

Taking Back the Month begins with a program that spans two menstrual cycles (roughly eight weeks). There are three basic starter plans for you to choose from: A "Basic PMS Plan" (for those who experience pain or somatic symptoms but no mood changes); a "Taming the Turmoil" plan (for those who experience anxiety, tension, irritability, and the like); and a "Banning the Blues" plan (for those whose symptoms gravitate toward depression, lethargy, teariness, and so on). Using one of the starter plans as a guide, you will discover how to develop your own plan of action, with specific activities for each week during the next two menstrual cycles. At the end of each menstrual cycle, you can review the steps you've been taking. By the end of the second cycle, you should have a pretty good idea of what works for you and whether some symptoms continue to be bothersome. At that point, you can add, delete, or modify particular treatment measures that you've tried.

Ideally, you should start with as many measures as you feel comfortable with for at least two months. Whichever ones you choose, every woman should begin by taking specific vitamin and mineral supplements—first, a multivitamin and mineral supplement during the postmenstrual phase of your cycle, then a PMS formula vitamin-mineral supplement during the premenstrual phase. Not only is this a good starting point—since swallowing a pill is relatively easy to do—but it may just jumpstart the relief process, making it easier for you to introduce other strategies. If you sense your own resistance to trying a particular strategy, think about why; the reason may tell you something about what's out of balance in your life. And that may persuade you more convincingly that you should try that particular strategy. In the UCSF PMS Symptom Management Program, women who found substantial relief from their symptoms used many different strategies from an average of three different categories (diet, exercise, relaxation, and so on). The combination of treatments that does the trick may vary considerably from one woman to the next.

Swinging into Action

Before getting started, spend some time setting priorities for the strategies you'd like to try. Ideally, schedule an hour to yourself and find a quiet place to map out your plan for the next two months. A few tools will make it easier to personalize your PMS solution.

The first is your **"PMS To-Do List,"** which will encompass your treatment goals, based on your individual symptoms, as well as specific steps within each treatment category (diet, exercise, relaxation, time management, and so on) that you'll use to achieve those goals. What you'll want to do is to look back over the goals you set at the end of chapters four through nine and list the treatment options you will start with now and state how frequently you will do it (daily, weekly, premenstrually, or as needed).

Regardless of your personal constellation of symptoms, every woman should start with the following priorities:

PMS TO-DO LIST

- **Supplements:** Take a daily multivitamin-mineral supplement from the first day of your period to midcycle; start taking a PMS-formula vitamin-mineral supplement each day from midcycle until the start of your next period.

- **Dietary changes:** Increase your daily water intake to four to six 8-ounce glasses postmenstrually and one to two quarts premenstrually; decrease your consumption of junk food and foods high in sugar and salt premenstrually.

- **Diet and physical activity evaluations:** Maintain a food and exercise diary postmenstrually and premenstrually (note: you'll find these in the Appendix).

- **Stress management:** Practice breathing and stretching exercises twice daily (even if it's only for five to ten minutes at a time).

- **Time management:** Analyze whether you're making the most of how you use your time; prioritize your premenstrual activities and identify stressful activities that may take longer than you think.

If your symptoms tend to belong to the "Turmoil" cluster, your overall priority will be to calm and control your mood, your behavior, and your physiological symptoms. To that end, you may want to add the following strategies to your "Taming the Turmoil To-Do List," in addition to following the basic priorities listed above:

- **Change diet to decrease stimulants. What to do:**

    Reduce intake of caffeine and simple sugars during the postmenstrual weeks and slash intake further premenstrually.

    Eat smaller, more frequent meals and snacks.

    Add protein-rich foods that are high in tryptophan.

- **Exercise to condition your body. What to do:**

    Increase physical activity during the day by taking the stairs, gardening, walking at lunchtime.

- **Relax to quiet the body and mind. What to do:**

    Practice progressive muscle relaxation (PMR) daily—for 20 to 30 minutes in the evening postmenstrually and for at least 30 minutes premenstrually.

    Add thought-stopping and thought-substitution strategies if you have trouble relaxing with PMR.

    Develop calming or comforting mental mini-vacations.

- **Use smart time-management tactics to reduce stress. What to do:**

    Practice saying "no" to non-essential requests and invitations.

    Delegate or eliminate unnecessary time-wasting activities.

    Block out time for PMS plan activities.

- **Identify sources of stress in your relationships. What to do:**

    Figure out who pushes your stress buttons and how you can prevent yourself from getting riled by those people.

    Assess your communication style.

Think about how you can use problem-solving strategies to solve interpersonal conflicts.

On the other hand, if your symptoms tend to congregate in "The Blues" cluster, your aim will to be revitalize and energize your lowered mood, compromised ability to function, and physical lethargy. To achieve these goals, in addition to following the advice from the basic list, your "Banning the Blues To-Do List" might look something like this:

- **Alter your diet to cultivate energy. What to do:**

  Eat small, frequent meals with complex carbohydrates to stabilize blood sugar and increase serotonin levels in the brain.

  Reduce alcohol intake all month but especially premenstrually.

  Eat more foods that are rich in magnesium, potassium, tyrosine, and tryptophan.

  Have a "Green Drink" or a potassium-rich smoothie in the morning or afternoon.

- **Exercise to rejuvenate your body. What to do:**

  Plan aerobic exercise for four to six times per week.

  Include an exercise class or a workout with a friend to make it social.

- **Use relaxation techniques to enhance mind-body vitality. What to do:**

  Practice autogenic training (AT) for 20 to 30 minutes daily for two weeks.

  Employ thought-stopping or -substitution strategies to banish negative thoughts.

  Develop revitalizing mental mini-vacations.

- **Carve out time for healthy activities. What to do:**

  Schedule daily activities—including sleep and awakening hours— in time blocks.

  Schedule time for PMS plan activities.

■ **Develop supportive social networks. What to do:**

Identify people in your home and work lives who support and inspire you.

Avoid people who drain your energy, especially in the premenstrual phase.

Develop direct, assertive communication skills.

THE PMS CALENDAR

Where to start? The PMS Plan Calendar, an 8-week calendar illustrated on pp. 166–169, will show you how to put your chosen plan into action, week by week. The Calendar is organized to start with the beginning of your next period. Depending on where you are in your cycle and how eager you are to launch your plan, you can wait until you get your period, you can start right now, or, if you happen to be premenstrual at the moment, you can start setting realistic goals and wait until your period arrives to get started. . . . The choice is up to you.

You have three options for choosing your starter plan for the PMS Calendar:

■ The Basic PMS Plan

■ The Taming the Turmoil Plan

■ The Banning the Blues Plan

Later, you can modify your treatment by consulting the "Symptom-Solution Section" that follows and provides specific advice on how to deal with symptoms such as breast tenderness, headaches, gastrointestinal discomfort, and sleep disturbances.

CUSTOMIZING YOUR PMS CALENDAR

After you've followed your chosen starter plan for a month or two, it's time to personalize it by adding specific strategies that will relieve your remaining premenstrual symptoms. By consulting the "Symptom-Solution Section" that follows, you'll discover what steps you can take to alleviate the particular discomfort you're continuing to experience.

By picking and choosing remedies that cater to your particular pre-menstrual problem, you will be developing a personalized plan of action that suits your needs. Once you've identified the solutions that make the most sense for you, it's time to customize your PMS calendar. Use a blank PMS Calendar ("My PMS Calendar" from page 170 or the Appendix) to develop your own plan. This should incorporate the strategies from the Basic PMS Plan, the Taming the Turmoil Plan, or the Banning the Blues Plan that you've already put into practice, as well as remedies that address the symptoms that remain after using your starter plan for a month or two. In other words, you'll continue to practice the must-do measures that you've begun to make a habit but you'll be supplementing these with additional strategies—or other symptom solutions—that are likely to help what's still bothering you.

Remember: Ultimately, you won't necessarily have to do all of these things all month long. It may just be three or four days a month where coffee or chocolate has a poisonous effect on you; or, it could be that you get the late-night jitters just two days before your period arrives. As you begin to monitor your cycle more closely, and as you begin to introduce some of these changes, you are likely to become highly attuned to the premenstrual shifts your body and mind experience—and to what you need to do to relieve the unpleasant ones. With practice, you might become so adept at a particular relaxation technique that you may be able to use it on an as-needed basis, rather than all month long. That's when you'll know that you've truly taken back the month.

PMS Plan Calendar: 8 Weeks
MONTH ONE

MONTH ONE	BASIC PLAN ACTIVITIES *Everyone starts with these activities*
WEEK 1: *The week your period arrives.*	▪ Begin taking a daily multiple vitamin and mineral supplement in the a.m. with juice and breakfast. ▪ Take 1,000 mg calcium at night with dinner. ▪ Keep a food diary (see Appendix) to determine where you might want to make changes. ▪ Increase water intake to at least one quart per day. ▪ Start relaxation activities: Schedule 5 minutes in the morning for breathing exercises and stretching and 5 minutes before bedtime. ▪ At the end of WEEK 1, make a reminder list of these activities and post it on your refrigerator.
WEEK 2: *POSTmenstrual week two*	▪ Continue with WEEK 1 activities and note any problems or questions that arise. ▪ Add thought-stopping exercises if you're having trouble clearing your mind during the relaxation exercises. ▪ Assess relationship stress: Reread communication style exercises. Think about a communication problem that recently occurred; rewrite the script. ▪ At the end of week 2, note any problems and what you might do to overcome them.
WEEK 3: *PREmenstrual week one*	▪ Stop taking the multivitamin-mineral and switch to the PMS formula vitamin-mineral supplement. Take daily for the next two weeks or through onset of next period. Divide recommended dose into 2 or 3 doses—morning, noon, and/or midafternoon—and take with a small amount of food or juice. Note effects in your PMS Notebook. ▪ Keep taking the calcium supplement at dinner- or bedtime with juice. ▪ Continue doing breathing exercises and stretching twice daily. ▪ Pay attention to your breathing during the day or when you feel stressed. Put "BREATHE" Post-it notes where needed.
WEEK 4: *PREmenstrual week two*	▪ Continue with WEEK 3 activities. ▪ Assess eating patterns and food cravings and how they change during premenstrual phase; note these in your food diary. ▪ Continue with PMS-formula vitamin-mineral supplement. Increase or decrease dose depending on effects. Continue taking calcium at night. ▪ Increase water intake to 1 to 2 quarts per day. ▪ Eat small, frequent snacks during the day or evening. Substitute complex carbohydrates for simple sugars. ▪ Record any new symptoms that begin as menstrual period approaches.

MONTH ONE

TAMING THE TURMOIL ACTIVITIES *Add these to calm your mood symptoms*	BANNING THE BLUES ACTIVITIES *Add these to revitalize your mood*
■ Reduce stimulants that aggravate turmoil symptoms: Reduce caffeine intake (1 cup coffee in morning is fine with low-fat milk or soy milk). Switch to juice or herbal teas in afternoon instead of colas or coffee. ■ Reduce your intake of simple sugars. ■ Try progressive muscle relaxation (PMR) and schedule time to practice daily.	■ Start the day with an energizing drink and some protein. ■ Schedule 5 minutes in a.m. to do energizing breathing exercises and stretching; 5 minutes of calming breathing and stretching before bedtime. ■ Choose an aerobic activity to do regularly and schedule exercise for five times per week even if it's for a short stint.
■ Analyze how you're spending your time if you are already feeling overwhelmed or having difficulty keeping up with your plan activities. ■ Practice saying "no" to unnecessary activities; block out 30 minutes each day for some PMS plan activity.	■ Try the autogenic training (AT) exercise or meditation. ■ Make a date with a close friend, family member, spouse, or partner to talk about your PMS plan and how they (or others) could help you with motivation, feedback, or support.
■ Reduce or eliminate caffeine premenstrually: Drink 1/2 cup of coffee in morning, no cola or black teas. ■ Drink no or very little alcohol this week. ■ Increase your water intake to nearly two quarts daily. Make Post-it note to remind yourself to drink every hour at work. ■ Rearrange your schedule to accommodate PMS: Look at what you need to do to prioritize activities or let go of stressful activities.	■ Eliminate alcohol during the week before your period. ■ Increase your intake of complex carbohydrates. ■ Write a revitalization mental mini-vacation and replay it when you feel the most fatigued or blue. ■ Identify toxic thoughts and cognitive distortions that you use the most; use thought-stopping and substitution exercises to banish them.
■ Assess your physical activity patterns, how they affect you, and which forms of exercise appeal to you; note these in your exercise diary. ■ Use breathing and calming strategies and/or take a time-out if you feel anxious, tense, and afraid that you'll say something you may later regret. ■ Say "no" when you need to avoid or delay a stressful situation.	■ Modify aerobic exercise if pain/discomfort symptoms are severe during this week. Try yoga on these days. ■ Write down a list of your strengths and keep them in your pocket; read it when you need a self-esteem boost. ■ Use relaxing or energizing breathing strategies if you feel tearful or unable to concentrate.

PMS Plan Calendar: 8 Weeks
MONTH TWO

MONTH ONE	BASIC PLAN ACTIVITIES *For everyone*
WEEK 5: *The week your* *period arrives.*	▪ Look at how the first cycle of your plan went. Consider what worked and what didn't work for you, your schedule, and your relationships. ▪ Start a new PMS Tracking Chart and record the same symptom list from the first month. ▪ Compare your post- and premenstrual diet and exercise patterns to help plan additional strategies. Establish new priorities in these areas. ▪ Continue WEEK 1 activities. ▪ Increase complex carbohydrates by adding more fruits and vegetables to each meal. ▪ Increase calcium supplement to 1,500 mg daily during the postmenstrual phase if you're getting little calcium from food. Stop taking the PMS-formula supplement and resume taking daily multivitamin.
WEEK 6: *POSTmenstrual* *week two*	▪ Continue with WEEK 5 activities. ▪ On exercise-free days, try yoga or stretching for 15 to 20 minutes at a time of day you like the best. If you have never done yoga before, get a book, rent or buy a videotape, or take an introductory class (see Appendix for resources). ▪ Evaluate your postmenstrual activities (WEEKS 1, 2, 5, and 6) and see what seems to be working. Note any problems and how you might overcome them.
WEEK 7: *PREmenstrual* *week one*	▪ Continue with WEEK 3 activities. ▪ Add more diet changes—increase your intake of complex carbohydrates and fiber; cut out premenstrual candy, sweets, salt, and salty foods. Keep small healthy meals/snacks on hand for ready access. ▪ Do breathing and stretching exercises twice daily or when you're feeling stressed or fatigued. ▪ Prioritize activities or reschedule stressful activities. Keep talking to your family, kids, and/or friends about helping with your personal PMS plan.
WEEK 8: *PREmenstrual* *week two*	▪ Continue with WEEK 4 and 7 activities. Note new symptoms or symptoms that are not decreasing in severity. See the "Symptom-Solution Section" that follows for additional strategies. ▪ Increase yoga exercises and/or substitute for walking if you're feeling fatigued or you have pain and discomfort. ▪ Evaluate your premenstrual activities (WEEKS 3, 4, 7, and 8) and consider what is working; note any problems and how to overcome them. ▪ Devise a schedule of activities for the postmenstrual and premenstrual weeks in the coming months.

MONTH TWO

TAMING THE TURMOIL ACTIVITIES *Calming activities*	BANNING THE BLUES ACTIVITIES *Revitalizing actions*
▪ Add a calming aerobic activity (such as walking, not Spinning). Set a realistic goal of walking for 20 to 30 minutes four days each postmenstrual week. Write this in your calendar as a reminder. ▪ Take a short walk at lunchtime; walk stairs instead of using the elevator; get up from your desk and stretch hourly. ▪ Practice PMR three times this week before bedtime or after work. ▪ Practice thought-stopping and thought-substitution exercises and combine with PMR to stop obsessing over worries.	▪ Increase your daily intake of fruits and vegetables and foods high in tyrosine and tryptophan. ▪ Eat foods that are high in magnesium and potassium. ▪ Schedule an energy-boosting snack to combat mid-afternoon fatigue. ▪ Use revitalizing breathing techniques before practicing AT. ▪ Develop a consistent wake-sleep schedule; avoid daytime naps. ▪ Use revitalizing mental mini-vacations or imagery to boost positive feelings.
▪ Schedule time for what matters including personal time and time for your PMS plan. ▪ Identify relationship problems and whether they're related to communication glitches or a conflict you haven't been willing to tackle. ▪ Plan a time to talk with your partner about your PMS plan. Ask for support and feedback.	▪ Evaluate the roles you fill and the people who increase your depressive feelings. Reduce the time you spend with these activities or people. ▪ Use time-blocking to organize daily activities and wake-sleep schedule. ▪ Schedule time with one or two friends to take a class (art, music, hiking).
▪ Do 20 to 30 minutes of PMR after work or before bed daily. ▪ Use thought-stopping exercises when your mind starts racing or negative self-talk gets in the way. ▪ Write out your worries, negative thoughts, or stresses rather than acting impulsively. ▪ Continue walking 3 to 4 times this week, or alternate walking with stretching or yoga.	▪ Do 20 to 30 minutes of AT before or after work daily. ▪ Use thought-stopping exercises when negative self-talk takes the microphone. ▪ Write about your negative thoughts or stresses instead of withdrawing into depression or sleep. ▪ Join an exercise class, bicycling group, or competitive sport to stay motivated.
▪ Reduce alcohol and caffeine all month long if you're noticing fewer turmoil symptoms. ▪ Check out the pattern of stress on your last PMS Tracking Chart. Look for correlations to symptoms. ▪ Write calming mental mini-vacations and use imagery during PMR practice. ▪ Evaluate the success of your PMS plan with your partner, spouse, or friend.	▪ Reduce alcohol all month long if you're experiencing less depression. ▪ Practice energizing mental mini-vacations and imagery during AT session. ▪ Look for a yoga class that incorporates energizing poses. ▪ Organize a self-help or PMS support group to help you continue making healthy changes.

My PMS Calendar

MONTH ONE	ACTIVITIES
WEEK 1: *(The week my period arrives.)*	■ Begin taking daily multiple vitamin-mineral supplement (with juice + breakfast). Take 1,000 mg. of calcium with dinner or at bedtime with juice. ■ Increase water intake to at least 1-qt. per day. ■ Do breathing-stretching exercises, 5 minutes twice a day. ■ ■ ■ At end of WEEK 1, make activity reminder list; post on refrigerator.
WEEK 2: *POSTmenstrual week two*	■ Continue WEEK 1 activities; note problems or questions. ■ ■ ■ ■ At end of WEEK 2, note problems and how to overcome them.
WEEK 3: *PREmenstrual week one*	■ STOP regular multis; SWITCH to PMS formula vitamin-mineral supplement. Take daily through onset of next period in 2 to 3 divided doses—morning, noon, and/or mid-afternoon. Continue taking calcium supplement. ■ Pay attention to breathing. Put "BREATHE" Post-it notes where needed. ■ ■ ■
WEEK 4: *PREmenstrual week two*	■ Continue WEEK 3 activities including PMS Tracking Chart. ■ Increase water to 1 to 2 quarts per day. ■ ■ ■ ■ ■ Record new symptoms that begin premenstrually.

MONTH TWO

MONTH TWO	ACTIVITIES
WEEK 5: *(The week my period arrives.)*	▪ Start new PMS Tracking Chart; continue WEEK 1 activities. ▪ ▪ ▪ ▪ ▪
WEEK 6: *POSTmenstrual week two*	▪ Continue WEEK 5 activities including PMS Tracking Chart. ▪ ▪ ▪ ▪
WEEK 7: *PREmenstrual week one*	▪ Continue with WEEK 3 activities. ▪ ▪ ▪ ▪ ▪
WEEK 8: *PREmenstrual week two*	▪ Continue with WEEK 4 and 7 activities. ▪ ▪ ▪ ▪ ▪ ▪

The Symptom-Solution Section

<u>PAIN, PAIN, GO AWAY . . .</u>

Body Aches and Pains

Many women experience musculoskeletal tenderness, stiffness, or pain in the back, neck, or joints during the premenstrual phase or their periods. This pain is not related to an underlying disorder, such as arthritis, or to a spine or joint malformation. It typically resolves by the end of a woman's period.

First-line treatment:

- Over-the-counter pain medications

  - Nonsteroidal anti-inflammatory drugs (NSAIDs), including aspirin, ibuprofen (Advil, Motrin), and naproxen (Aleve, Anaprox), will reduce the intensity of pain and reduce inflammation. Start with a larger dose—two to three tablets every five to six hours—for the first couple of days of pain, then decrease the dosage to one to two tablets three or four times daily until your period begins. If you also have menstrual cramps, continue this dosage schedule during your period.
  - Capsaicin creams have been found to produce a gradual decrease in joint pain and stiffness if they're applied three to five times per day. Capsaicin, a component of chili peppers, blocks the biochemicals of pain.

- Try a heating pad or soaking in a hot bath for about 30 minutes to increase blood flow to the muscles. You can now buy 12-hour heat pads with special fittings for the neck, back, knee, and lower abdomen.

- Avoid physically demanding activities for a few days; substitute stretching or gentle yoga for high-impact exercise. (See Chapter Five for stretching exercises.)

If pain and discomfort persist:

- Perform stretching exercises for the neck and back two to three times per day; move slowly and do not stretch beyond the point of pain. Stop any activity that hurts. (See Chapter five for more information.)

- If you notice increased pain and stiffness after sleeping, you may want to add extra cushioning to your mattress or change your sleeping position so that you're lying on your side or back with your knees and neck supported by pillows.

- Take short rest periods throughout the day to ease pressure on your back, neck, and joints. Lie down, support your neck with a pillow, and place a pillow under your knees.

Prevention strategies:

- Pay attention to your posture—including how you sit, stand, and carry items—and try to reduce the strain on your spine and neck. When standing, keep your neck straight, your head held high, your pelvis forward, and your abdomen and buttocks tucked in. When sitting, keep your spine against the back of your chair and your knees a little higher than your hips. When carrying items, remember that heavy purses and briefcases can put pressure on your back; try to alter the load or use a backpack.

- Perform low-impact exercise regularly, as well as stretching routines, to condition your back, joints, and muscles. Over time, this will also help decrease premenstrual musculoskeletal pain and discomfort. If you have regular, but not severe, back and neck pain that don't come and go with your menstrual cycle, consult a physical therapist for an evaluation and recommedations for back-strengthening exercises.

Breast Swelling and Tenderness

Breast swelling and pain that occur one to two weeks before the start of your period are normal responses to fluctuating hormone levels. But that doesn't mean sore breasts aren't annoying. These symptoms may become more intense during the perimenopausal transition but they generally disappear after menopause when ovarian hormones stabilize at a lower level.

First-line treatment:

■ Take a nonprescription pain reliever such as acetaminophen (Tylenol) or one of the NSAIDs (aspirin, ibuprofen, and the like).

■ Wear a comfortable and supportive bra, especially while exercising—one that does not irritate the nipple area as you move.

■ Consider trying a nutritional remedy. Most of these have yielded mixed results in research but some women find relief from one or more of the following strategies:

  • Eliminate or dramatically cut back on caffeine from all sources.
  • Take 400–800 IU of vitamin E daily.
  • Consume omega-3 and omega-6 fatty acids (see the Cramps section for recommended dosage).
  • Reduce your salt intake to reduce fluid retention. (See Chapter Four for more information.)

Prevention strategies:

■ Talk to your health-care practitioner about whether you're a candidate for oral contraceptives. These quiet the body's naturally occurring hormonal effects on the breast, although the first couple of months on the Pill may increase breast tenderness. Keep in mind: Finding the right pill for you is a matter of trial and error. (See Chapter Twelve for more information.)

Cramps

Premenstrual or menstrual cramps (a.k.a., dysmenorrhea) are thought to be due to the release of prostaglandins, the hormones that stimulate contractions of the uterus. In women who experience these cramps, it may be that prostaglandins are produced in excess—or that they're particularly sensitive to them. Either way, pain can occur in the abdomen, pelvic region, the back, or the thighs.

First-line treatment:

■ Consider taking one of the nonsteroidal anti-inflammatory drugs (NSAIDs), which inhibit the production of prostaglandins. NSAIDs are available as prescription versions—higher doses of naproxen (e.g., Anaprox, Naproxyn), ibuprofen (e.g., prescription-strength Motrin), and others (such as ketoprofen) as well as the new COX-2 inhibitors such as Celebrex or Vioxx—as well as in over-the-counter (OTC) doses in the form of ibuprofen (such as Advil, Motrin, or Nuprin) and naproxen (e.g., Aleve). Aceta-minophen is not an NSAID, but some women find that it relieves the backaches that are often associated with menstrual cramps.

Keep in mind that the timing and strength of the dose are critical to pain relief. Take the medication at the first twinge of pain or before bleeding occurs at an adequate dose. You might take two ibuprofen tablets three to four times per day for the first three days of your period. Or, you could take two tablets of naproxen for your initial (or loading) dose, followed by one to two tablets two to three times daily for the first three days of your period. (Of course, feel free to keep up this regimen if pain persists for more than three days but don't take these drugs for more than several days because they can increase gastrointestinal distress.)

- Apply heat with a hot water bottle or a heating pad, or immerse yourself in a hot bath. Continuously applying topical heat to treat dysmenorrhea initiates relaxation of the smooth muscles and decreases pain perception. If you want to use the latest incarnation of the old-fashioned hot-water bottle, you can purchase Thermacare™, a disposable pad that's shaped for the abdomen and can be worn under clothing.

If pain and discomfort persist:
- Increase your intake of essential fatty acids such as linoleic acid (omega-3 fatty acids) and gamma linolenic acid (GLA or omega-6 fatty acid). Omega-3 fatty acids, found in fish oil, have been found to relieve painful periods and GLA can ease premenstrual breast tenderness, pelvic cramps, and fluid retention. You can take fish oil capsules or increase your intake of fish. If you decide to go the supplement route, look for a commercial preparation that contains 1,000 mg. of EPA (eicosapentaenoic acid)—and 700 mg. of DHA (docosahexaenoic acid)—and take it daily for two months in one or two divided doses. For optimal absorption, these essential fatty acids require that vitamin E (approximately 400 I.U.) be taken along with them; check the

amount of vitamin E in your regular multivitamin and mineral supplement as well as your PMS formula supplement before adding more. (See Chapter Eleven for more information.)

- Try evening primrose oil, which is a dietary source of GLA, if cyclical pelvic pain and breast tenderness persist after using omega-3 fatty acids for one to two months. You can ingest 2,000 to 3,000 mg. of evening primrose oil capsules daily. (See Chapter Eleven for more information.)

- Get a massage. Both Swedish and Oriental massage can relieve pain and muscle tension, including the discomfort of premenstrual cramping. (See Chapter Eleven for more information.)

- Put a buzz on the pain. Transcutaneous electrical nerve stimulation (TENS) can provide relief for pelvic pain either by itself or in combination with NSAIDs. TENS requires a handheld device with small electrodes that attach to areas of the body (such as the abdomen and lower back) that hurt; the device delivers a small electrical pulse that disrupts the sensory perception of pain, thereby short-circuiting the experience of pain.

- Talk to your health-care practitioner about whether you're a candidate for oral contraceptives. Oral contraceptives are effective at regulating the menstrual cycle and reducing the volume of menstrual fluid and circulating prostaglandins; these changes can, in turn, decrease menstrual pain. Monophasic or triphasic low-estrogen oral contraceptives are equally effective, in this respect.

- Consult your health-care provider. If, after trying all these measures, your pain continues to be debilitating, you may have an underlying pelvic or uterine problem. In that case, you will require medical evaluation by a specialist in gynecology.

Headaches

One of the most common symptoms, whether they're associated with the menstrual cycle or not, headaches come in many different varieties. The tension-type is usually characterized by dull, steady pain across the head and neck. The migraine type often involves throbbing, pulsating pain, in addition to visual disturbances, light sensitivity, nausea, vomiting, and sinus symptoms that may last from a few hours to days. And the cluster variety, which is more common in men, is marked by severe, piercing pain that's located on one side of the head or over one eye; these can last anywhere from a few minutes to hours.

First-line treatment:
- Start with an OTC pain reliever, such as aspirin, acetaminophen, or a nonsteroidal anti-inflammatory drug (NSAID) like ibuprofen (Advil or Nuprin, for example). If it's a migraine, drink a small amount of caffeine after taking a pain reliever; or take extra strength Excedrin, which contains caffeine as well as pain-relieving medication.

- Sit or lie down in a dark, quiet room and try to relax for 20 to 30 minutes. Place an ice pack on your forehead and neck. Tension headaches sometimes respond better to the application of heat. Try whichever temperature appeals to you.

Prevention strategies:
- Track your headaches and try to pinpoint the factors that trigger them. Typical tension headache triggers include stress, fatigue, too much sleep, activities that require repetitive motion, chewing gum or grinding your teeth, and lack of body conditioning. Migraine headaches can be hormonally triggered before or during menstruation, during pregnancy, the perimenopause, or with the use of oral contraceptives. Non-cyclical migraines occur randomly although they can be triggered by certain foods and beverages (tyramine-containing foods, chocolate, nuts, smoked fish, cured meats, aged cheeses, MSG, and red wine, to name a few), lack of sleep, bright lights, weather changes, stress, and strong odors. If you can identify your triggers, you may be able to avoid some of them; if you can't, knowing what factors increase your vulnerability can alert you to signs of a budding headache.

- Learn to relax. By reducing muscle tension and your perception of stress, you may be able to head off a fair number of headaches. (See Chapter Six for relaxation strategies.)

- Move your body on a regular basis. Doing regular aerobic exercise, improving your posture, and doing regular muscle stretching exercises, concentrating on the head, neck, and shoulders, can prevent tension headaches. (See Chapter Five for exercise details.)

■ Treat yourself to a massage. Whether it's a traditional massage or acupressure, releasing physical tension and improving circulation can promote feelings of well-being—and perhaps prevent tension-type headaches. (See Chapter Eleven for more information.)

If headaches persist:

■ Get evaluated by a health-care practitioner who specializes in headache diagnosis and treatment if migraines are severe or don't respond to these measures. There are prescription medications that are safe and effective. Some menstrually related migraines respond to ovarian suppression with oral contraceptives. If you are sure your headache is a migraine-type, therapies such as acupuncture and biofeedback can also be effective.

■ Don't ignore incapacitating headaches. Sometimes a headache is a symptom of an underlying problem—either physical or psychological. If you have tried various treatments or your headaches become more intense or persistent, consult a medical or mental health professional for further diagnosis and evaluation.

SOOTHING MEASURES FOR BODY AND MIND

Bloating

The surge of hormones that occurs just before your period can cause your kidneys to retain salt and water. As a result, you may feel bloated in your belly. Your fingers, ankles, and feet may be swollen. And the area beneath your eyes may appear puffy. It's temporary water weight—but it's annoying, nonetheless.

First-line treatment:

■ Consume foods that naturally decrease fluid retention. These include:

- Asparagus—lightly cooked or steamed.
- Apple cider vinegar—sprinkle 1 tablespoon on a salad or drink it by diluting with a small amount of water.

- Alfalfa sprouts or dandelion flowers—add to salads.
- A handful of dandelion greens blended with 2 celery stalks and 4 carrots into a juice.
- Dandelion or alfalfa leaf tea: Steep 1 to 2 teaspoons of the dried leaves in a cup of water for 10 minutes; drink up to 3 cups per day.
- Add 2 parts burdock root (a mild diuretic) to 2 parts dandelion greens to make about ¼ cup of the herb mixture. Mix this with a quart of cold water and simmer at a low boil for 15 minutes; cool, strain, and drink 3 to 4 cups of tea during the day for severe fluid retention.
- If you use these, make sure to also increase your potassium intake (cantaloupe, bananas, apricots, black beans, lentils, potatoes, and other good sources mentioned in Chapter Four).

- Get physical. Moderate to vigorous aerobic exercise will make you sweat—and hasten the transport of water through your body. (See Chapter Five for more information.)

- Elevate your feet if you're prone to swelling in the legs. And wear supportive stockings to alleviate discomfort.

- See the section on gastrointestinal symptoms if bloating is due to constipation.

Digestive Distress: Diarrhea and Constipation

Some women experience diarrhea, constipation, or alternating bouts of each during the week before or the first few days of their period. Once you have established a balanced, whole-grain diet, these gastrointestinal symptoms are likely to diminish as the healthy, rhythmic contractions of the digestive tract are re-established.

First-line treatment:

- Increase fiber in your diet for diarrhea and constipation that is limited to the premenstrual period. You can do this by adding bran cereal, whole grains, rice bran, nuts, vegetables, and fruit to your meals. In the morning, you can add psyllium (Metamucil is a brand form) to fruit juice. This creates bulk in the intestines and soaks up toxins and gas to ensure regular motility of the intestines and regular bowel movements, which will result in decreased intestinal cramps, diarrhea, and constipation.

■ Make sure that you drink at least 16 ounces of water with a bulking agent like psyllium or Metamucil. Drinking hot water with lemon juice will also stimulate motility in the morning.

■ Stop diarrhea by chewing 1 tablespoon of dried blueberries and wash them down with water; they act as an astringent to pucker up the bowel, according to the late Varro Tyler, Ph.D., author of *The Honest Herbal*.

■ Avoid alcohol, caffeine, milk, and dairy products as well as artificial sweeteners until diarrhea has subsided. Instead, follow the BRAT diet—bananas, rice, applesauce, and toast—until your intestines start behaving properly.

■ Add an electrolyte drink (such as Gatorade or EmergenC powder) and eat potassium-rich foods to restore the balance of electrolytes in your body, after a bout of diarrhea. You can also use yogurt or acidophilus capsules to replace normal lactobacillus in the intestines.

■ Avoid antidiarrheal medications for a day or two until you have given these other remedies a chance to work.

If constipation or diarrhea persist:

■ Retrain your intestines. Chew your food slowly and thoroughly to activate salivary and stomach enzymes. Try to have a regular time for a bowel movement. Don't wait if you have the urge.

■ Consume lots of fiber (including psyllium) and water all month long if you have a chronic problem with constipation. If you continue to experience constipation, add magnesium to your diet— by taking 200 mg. of a magnesium oxide or magnesium citrate supplement at bedtime. Don't worry: This will not create a laxative dependency.

■ Drink an oral rehydration solution—available at drug stores—if you experience persistent, watery diarrhea in spite of these remedies. Have one to two cups for every episode of diarrhea. Sports drinks, such as Gatorade, are a second choice because they do not usually contain enough sodium or potassium to be useful; also, their high sugar content may aggravate the diarrhea. If you don't have a fever and the diarrhea slows but doesn't go away, you can later take an OTC antidiarrheal remedy such as Pepto-Bismol (bismuth subsalicylate), Immodium (loperamide), or Lomotil (diphenoxylate hydrochloride).

- Consult your primary care provider if you have a fever, if you notice blood in your stool, or if diarrhea increases. Likewise, if intestinal cramping and gas persist all month in spite of these remedies, you may have irritable bowel syndrome or another disorder that requires medical attention.

Indigestion, Nausea

Indigestion includes symptoms of heartburn, gas, belching, and intestinal cramping; in persistent form, it is sometimes referred to as gastroesophageal reflux disease (GERD, for short). If these symptoms occur exclusively during the premenstrual phase, they are probably related to increased gastrointestinal movement. Nausea may also be a part of the premenstrual gastrointestinal upset and discomfort or it may be associated with a stress reaction.

First-line treatment:
- Start with the general recommendations under the constipation and diarrhea section.

- Drink chamomile tea made from 2 to 4 teaspoons of chamomile flower heads, steeped in 1 cup of boiling water, three times a day.

- Make yourself a GI-calming "green drink." (See Chapter Four for the recipe.)

- If you're not taking a PMS formula supplement, take a B-complex vitamin that contains 50 mg. of B-6 to quell nausea.

- Have some ginger to ease nausea. Swallow a ginger capsule (which contains 500 mg. per pill) or brew a ginger tea (2 teaspoons of powdered or grated ginger root per cup of water). If you have diabetes or a heart condition, do not take high doses of ginger on a daily basis.

- OTC antihistamines, such as Benadryl or Dramamine, can be taken for premenstrual nausea, though they will make you sleepy. Take these for no longer than a few days and drink plenty of water.

- Apply pressure. Acupressure has been found to be effective for reducing nausea and motion sickness. You can purchase acupressure wrist bands in many pharmacies.

If indigestion persists:

- Drink a "green drink" every morning.

- Avoid conflict during meals. Start with a few deep cleansing breaths before beginning a meal and make sure you continue to breathe fully while you eat.

- Eat low-fat, low-sugar yogurt or acidophilus milk as a snack; you can also supplement with acidophilus capsules.

- Brew a cup of licorice root tea and drink it two to three times per day. This herb has been found to be as effective as an antacid. Or, you can take a nonprescription liquid antacid at one hour and again at three hours after meals and again at bedtime.

- Digestive enzyme formulas made from fruit and vegetables are available in capsules at health-food stores and can be taken daily.

Fatigue

Whether it occurs with or without mood changes, a feeling of being bone-tired strikes many women for a few days before their periods. Or, they may experience more mild fatigue throughout the premenstrual phase. Or they may feel as though they simply don't have their usual stamina. Without a doubt, it can be difficult to function normally under these conditions.

First-line treatment:

- If you feel sleepy and lethargic after a meal that's high in starchy carbohydrates—pancakes or pasta, for instance—balance out the carbohydrate load with some low-fat protein (low-fat yogurt, cottage cheese, tuna or other fish, beans, or lentils).

- Eat low-fat protein snacks—soy, low-fat cheeses, and reduced-fat peanut butter—as well as foods that alkalinize the body (most fruits and vegetables).

- Increase your intake of plant-based foods that are high in potassium and magnesium. (See Chapter Four for details.)

- Try autogenic training to revitalize your mind and body; write an energizing mental mini-vacation and combine this with relaxation practice. (See Chapter Six for more information.)

- Start exercising aerobically for 15-minute sessions three to four times per week. Practice yoga exercises that are energizing or the rejuvenating breath. (See Chapter Six for more information.)

If fatigue persists:
- Add a potassium and a magnesium supplement if you're not taking a PMS-formula supplement.

- See your health-care provider if you're exhausted all month. It could be that an underlying health condition or a medication you're taking is making you tired all the time.

Skin Disorder Flare-ups

Dermatitis or eczema, both of which cause itching, can occur premenstrually or perimenopausally due to a predominance of progesterone which stimulates oil production in the skin. Itching typically occurs on the hands, wrists, face, scalp, behind the knees, and inside the elbows, and it can increase with mounting stress. If you are sure that the itching is not due to an irritant or underlying condition, some remedies to stop the vicious itch-scratch cycle can reduce discomfort.

First-line treatment:
- Control itching by using an OTC topical cortisone cream or lotion or a Calamine-type lotion. Oral antihistamines, taken at bedtime, can relieve the itching sensation, making it easier for you to sleep.

- Calm itching by applying cool compresses or a washcloth that's been soaked in milk mixed with water. Or, make a strong tea with chamomile flower heads, allow it to cool, then apply it to the skin with a soft cloth.

- Place 1 to 2 cups of baking soda into a lukewarm bath and soak for about 30 minutes. Afterwards, pat yourself dry; don't rub your skin with a towel.

- Talk yourself out of scratching and use breathing and relaxation strategies to resist the urge. Also, keep your fingernails short, smooth, and clean.

If itching persists:
- See your health-care provider if the itching doesn't respond to these measures and drives you mad; or if it continues beyond the premenstrual period. It could be due to an underlying health condition or an allergic reaction.

Acne Breakouts
Facial blackheads, whiteheads, pustules, and cysts often occur or worsen during the premenstrual phase, even in grown women. Pimples can also pop up on the back, neck, and buttocks in adolescents. Although there is no known cure for acne—premenstrual or otherwise—some remedies can keep these blemishes under control.

First-line treatment:
- Increase your water intake and try to get more rest to promote waste excretion and restoration of various body systems.

- Increase your intake of foods that are high in beta-carotene—carrots, pumpkin, cantaloupe, and other yellow-orange fruits and vegetables—to promote healthy skin. While there is no known relationship between specific foods and acne flare-ups, if you notice your own personal dietary triggers for acne, avoid those foods.

- Keep your hair and face extra clean. Wash your face with a non-oily soap or lotion—don't scrub!—and avoid hot steam or facial saunas as these can aggravate acne. Wash your hands frequently and don't touch your face. Also, avoid greasy hair creams and keep your hair away from your face while you sleep. If you wear a sweatband or headband during exercise, wash these often in hot water to avoid letting the sweat buildup promote acne.

- Apply a benzoyl peroxide solution (with a 5 to 10 percent concentration, depending on your skin's sensitivity); these are available in lotion, gel, or cream form and help to loosen the skin's oil plugs. If you're prone to acne, use only water-based makeup and tread lightly with moisturizing lotion. Be sure to thoroughly remove all makeup before turning in for the night.

- Practice yoga. Selected yoga poses can increase blood flow to the face.

If acne persists:
- Increase your intake of omega-6 fatty acids in the form of black currant seed oil or evening primrose oil. Take three 500 mg. capsules daily for three months.

- Avoid prolonged exposure to the sun. While sun and UV lamps may dry up acne, they also cause long-term skin damage so it's best to steer clear of these as much as possible.

- See your health-care provider. If acne does not resolve after your period, or if you have enlarged, tender lymph nodes, you may have a bacterial skin infection that requires antibiotic treatment.

Forgetfulness and Difficulty Concentrating

These symptoms may be related to fluid retention, stress, lack of sleep, or too much sleep. They are usually short-lived and decrease with the implementation of the PMS plan.

First-line treatment:
- Review the "Taming the Turmoil" and "Banning the Blues" plans, earlier in this chapter, if you suspect your lack of concentration is related to anxiety and feeling out of control or to fatigue and depression. (You'll find more stress-management strategies in Chapter Six.)

- Check out the sleep remedies that follow in this section if you are having trouble sleeping. Memory and cognitive symptoms could be related.

- Reduce your intake of saturated fats by increasing your consumption of plant-based proteins.

- Eat lots of fruits and vegetables to increase your consumption of natural antioxidants.

- Make sure that your daily multivitamin and mineral supplement includes iron. Low levels of iron can be associated with memory problems.

- Increase your intake of omega-3 fatty acids by eating fish two to three times per week and by taking 100 to 400 IU of vitamin E daily.

Prevention strategies:
- Practice yoga and meditation to help improve concentration and cognitive alertness. (See Chapters Six and Seven for details.) While you are doing your yoga workout or relaxation exercises, you can silently and slowly count backward from 100 once you are in a relaxed state or yoga pose. As your concentration improves, start back from 200 or 500. This will help stimulate circuitry in the brain.

- Think about taking gingko biloba. The herb seems to help reverse memory loss by increasing blood circulation to the brain, according to the late herb expert Varro Tyler, Ph.D. If you take a gingko supplement, be sure to follow the directions on the product's label. And keep in mind: Herbs, unlike drugs, generally take a few weeks of daily use to create improvement.

- If symptoms persist, talk with your health-care provider about checking your hemoglobin levels; you may be anemic and need more than just iron therapy.

Night Sweats and Hot Flashes

If these occur for a couple of days right before or during menstruation, don't worry: It doesn't mean you are entering the perimenopausal transition. Yes, it's the same experience as the legendary menopausal symptoms but in a milder version during the premenstrual phase. Body temperature changes can be stimulated by the drop in ovarian hormones just before the onset of the menstrual period.

First-line treatment:
- Avoid alcohol, spicy foods, and hot baths to minimize additional hot flash triggers if you notice these symptoms every menstrual cycle, and they are uncomfortable.

- Check out the remedies for sleep problems (in the section that follows) if hot flashes and night sweats are interfering with your sleep. This often happens as women enter their forties: At this stage, hot flashes and night sweats are probably occurring along with irregular periods and are likely to be related to a change in ovarian function. (See Chapters Eleven and Twelve for alternative and pharmacological strategies.)

If night sweats and hot flashes persist:
- If hot flashes and night sweats increase in frequency and intensity, whether or not they are related to the perimenopause, consult your health-care provider.

When the World Seems Topsy Turvy

Dizziness, a rapid heartbeat, or heart palpitations may be due to over-activity of the vagus nerve, which is part of the autonomic nervous system. The vagus nerve lies next to the intestines and controls the heart, intestines, and the circulatory system. This nerve can be stimulated by a heightened stress response, panic attacks, premenstrual or perimenopausal changes in ovarian hormones, as well as prolonged standing (due to the pooling of blood in the legs).

First-line treatment:
- Check your heart rate by feeling your pulse, at your wrist or neck, to determine if your heart rhythm is actually increased. If your heart rate is higher than normal (greater than 90 beats per minute) then you may have an underlying medical condition that needs attention.

- Decrease your intake of stimulants such as caffeine, nicotine, and sugar. (See Chapter Four for more information.)

- Regularly perform slow, deep breathing exercises and forward stretching exercises in a seated position to avoid falling. (See Chapters Five and Six for details.)

- Practice relaxation strategies—either PMR or AT—to calm your physiological response. (See Chapter Six for more information.)

If dizziness or heart palpitations persist:
- If these symptoms do not respond to the previous measures, see a health professional. If you experience dizziness that is not related to a stress reaction or that occurs at other times of the month than the premenstrual phase, you may have an underlying medical condition. These symptoms could be related to anemia (if you have heavy periods or a history of anemia, you may want to have a complete blood count or hematocrit blood test); or, they could be related to low blood pressure, low blood sugar levels, or a thyroid disorder.

RECLAIMING CONTROL OF YOUR FACULTIES

Sleep Havoc
Whether you struggle with falling asleep, staying asleep, waking up too early, or sleeping too much, you may be able to regain snooze control with some basic sleep-hygiene strategies. These include sticking with a regular sleep-wake pattern, maintaining bedtime rituals and routines, avoiding or minimizing food and alcohol before bed, getting daily exercise and exposure to bright daytime light, and creating an optimal environment for sleep.

First-line treatment:
- Avoid large meals and alcohol late in the evening or before bedtime; nicotine can cause wakefulness, too.

- Practice relaxation activities for 20 to 30 minutes before bedtime to reduce muscle tension; other activities conducive to relaxation include reading, listening to music, or taking a warm bath.

- Get up and go to another room if you're unable to fall asleep or return to sleep easily. The reason: You want to associate your bed with sleep, not being unable to sleep. If you do stay in bed, practice relaxation, calming, or meditation strategies to help ease yourself into slumber.

- Drink an herbal tea containing valerian root; it is a natural sleep aid with proven benefits. Valerian has no known toxicity and is not habit-forming. Many women find it helps them fall asleep faster and stay asleep longer.

- If you use a sleep medication—whether prescription or nonprescription—do not use it for more than three days. Otherwise, you could build up a tolerance to the drug or wreak havoc on the natural stages of your sleep.

- Eat melatonin-rich foods such as oats, sweet corn, rice, ginger, tomatoes, and bananas. Melatonin, sold as a dietary supplement, is really an unregulated hormonal drug but some people find that taking 1 to 3 mg. 30 minutes before bedtime is helpful.

Prevention strategies:
- Plan aerobic or intense exercise earlier in the day. For the sake of slumber quality, try to avoid exercising within three or four hours of bedtime.

- Use the bed and bedroom only for sleep and sex, not for working, paying bills, or watching TV.

- Avoid daytime naps. Even short naps at varying times of the day can result in more fragmented sleep and insomnia at night.

- Decrease your exposure to bright nighttime light. You may need to light-proof your bedroom with blackout shades or wear eye shades. Also, don't spend much time in a brightly lit bathroom before turning in; otherwise, you may inadvertently upset your body's internal clock, reducing and delaying the secretion of sleep-inducing melatonin.

- Stick with a regular sleep-wake schedule. Your body's internal clock craves consistency and predictability. Establish a regular bedtime and time to rise in the morning. Set an alarm and don't hit the snooze button, regardless of how you slept the previous night.

Food Cravings or Bingeing

Premenstrual hormonal changes—as well as the other physiological shifts that are set into motion—can trigger food cravings, increased appetite, and/or overeating in some women. This is often the most difficult time to exercise dietary restraint, especially when it comes to sweet or salty foods or alcohol. (In fact, women who have eating disorders or who abuse alcohol often experience a worsening of their disorders during the period before their period.)

First-line treatment:

- Increase your intake of water and juices that are high in vitamin C (citrus, vegetable, and tomato, for example). Also, consume potassium-rich foods (such as bananas, apricots, black beans, lentils, and potatoes) when you experience cravings. (See Chapter Four for more recommendations.)

- Put yourself in a calmer state. Engaging in meditation or relaxation exercises during the times that you experience cravings can help you resist acting on your cravings or bingeing. Before you start, drink a glass of water and have a small protein- or complex carbohydrate–rich snack. (See Chapter Seven for relaxation exercises.)

If cravings or bingeing persist:

- Seek help. If overeating or bingeing on food or alcohol is or becomes a constant problem, you may want to consider joining a structured or supervised weight control or dietary program. Or you may have an eating disorder or alcohol abuse problem that requires professional treatment.

Angry Outbursts

Learning to deal with anger can be challenging for men and women—at any time of the month. As with many stress-related responses, angry outbursts may have become a knee-jerk reaction, one in which you lash out at the person who upsets you. Anger management involves paying attention to provocational or situational triggers and developing skills that will help you handle conflicts more constructively. The first step is to change your cognitive approach to the expression of premenstrual anger—to remind yourself that you do have some control over yourself, despite how you're feeling.

First-line treatment:

- Question your motives. In situations where you feel your blood boiling, Redford Williams, M.D., author of *Anger Kills*, recommends asking yourself the following questions before reacting impulsively: Is the situation important to me? Is my reaction appropriate based on the facts? Is there anything I can do to modify or change the situation?

    If you answer "no" to any of these questions, then it's time to use your breathing, relaxation, or meditation techniques and chill out. Save your energy for something that you can do something about. (See Chapter Six for relaxation strategies.)

    If your answer is "yes" to all of these questions, then ask yourself, "Would it be worth it, given the situation, to take action?" If so, then act, but in a calm, proactive way or delay acting until you can come up with a better, long-term solution.

- Do what doesn't come naturally. When you are feeling angry and are having trouble controlling your tongue, try to defuse the anger by confronting someone calmly but firmly or by doing something to make yourself feel better.

- Don't try to reason with an angry person. It just doesn't work. Instead, control your own temper but let the other person know that you won't talk to him or her until he or she has calmed down and will treat you with respect. When you get back together, use the communication and problem-solving strategies in Chapter Nine to help you resolve the conflict successfully.

- Put yourself in the other person's shoes. Think about why the other person is angry. Or think about all the different ways that you can view the situation. Viewing situations in a more positive or neutral light can help you nip anger in the bud and take a more constructive approach to addressing the underlying issues.

Prevention strategies:

- Explore your past experiences with anger by writing in a journal. Analyze your anger by rating it on a ten-point scale, based on the

intensity, how long it lasts, and the short- and long-term consequences of your hostile feelings. This will help you to see patterns
to your feelings and behavior. Explore how anger has damaged
personal relationships, created difficulties at work, or embarrassed you in social situations. Then think about how you can
develop other ways of thinking or behaving in anger-evoking situations. Or, try to find a role model who handles difficult situations gracefully and look at how that person copes with
frustration and tension.

- Desensitize your angry responses by using the thought-stopping
  exercise. Use your relaxation time to recall a situation where you
  erupted in anger. Once you have let the memory activate your
  mind, use deep-breathing and progressive muscle relaxation or
  other relaxation techniques to calm the tension in your body. This
  process allows you to defuse your anger reaction automatically.

- Be forgiving of yourself if you don't control your anger all of the
  time. Setbacks are common with the effort to overcome any bad
  habit. What's important is to take responsibility for the slipup,
  learn from the experience, and continue making progress.

- Compare notes with your spouse. It's likely that the two of you
  have performed the anger cha-cha together, with one person triggering the other's ire. If you can both be committed to reducing
  conflict in your relationship, it will be that much easier to choose
  another communicative dance.

If angry outbursts persist:
- Consider seeking professional help if you or your partner find it
  impossible to control angry outbursts or they become more frequent and intense. Likewise, if your anger is threatening your
  relationships and your self-esteem, your career progress, or your
  health. Sometimes, anger is related to an underlying depression
  or psychiatric disorder and medication can be helpful.

GRADE YOUR OWN REPORT CARD

After you've completed month two or three of your PMS plan,
depending on how quickly you've swung into action, it will be time to

evaluate how well your plan is working. Before going any further, give yourself a pat on the back for the considerable effort you've made to revamp your habits—and for the strides you've made so far. Once you've paused to congratulate yourself, it's time to consider what's next. Start by thinking globally about how you're feeling. Overall, have your premenstrual symptoms eased in severity? Did your stress levels go down while you were following the plan? Did your sense of well-being rise?

To find out the true answers to these questions, compare your "PMS Tracking Charts" from the first month to the second or third month after implementing your plan. Which symptoms disappeared altogether? Which symptoms decreased in severity? Which symptoms are still bothering you? Record this information in the appropriate columns on the "Before and After Chart" that follows. This will give you an unvarnished look at how your plan is succeeding and where there's room for improvement.

After you've identified the remaining symptoms, it's time, once again, to set priorities for how you'll address them. Look back at the treatment advice that corresponds to your still-present symptoms and see what you haven't tried yet. You can read about these strategies in the "Symptom-Solution Section," as well as in the previous chapters, then set specific priorities for the strategies you'd like to try next. Write these down on the lower half of your "Before and After Chart."

Before and After Chart

Compare your symptoms from the first (pretreatment) PMS Tracking Chart with your symptoms from the first or second treatment month and answer the following questions:

Which symptoms have gone away completely?	Which symptoms have decreased in severity?	Which symptoms remain?
1._____	1._____	1._____
2._____	2._____	2._____
3._____	3._____	3._____
4._____	4._____	4._____
5._____	5._____	5._____

Your New PMS To-Do List:
Depending on the remaining symptoms or those that you still want to try to reduce in severity, revise your original To-Do list here.

1. _____

2. _____

3. _____

4. _____

5. _____

6. _____

Now it's time to establish your long-term PMS plan. What you'll want to do is to fill out a new PMS chart—the "Getting On With Life Blueprint," which follows—with the strategies you've been using week by week as well as the new ones you plan to try next. We've provided the basic must-do measures that every woman with PMS should practice but beyond that, you're on your own. It's up to you to establish a schedule of steps and activities that make sense for your symptoms and your life. Some you might do all month long; others you might do just during the premenstrual phase. For this reason, you really need to give some thought to what measures have helped at certain times of the month and how you could best use your time to enhance your health and well-being. In the "Blueprint" framework that's provided, the must-do measures are spelled out and the plan is divided into postmenstrual weeks and premenstrual weeks; beyond this, you'll find categories of strategies (Diet, Exercise, Relaxation, Thought-Changing, and so on) to help you organize your chosen activities. The selections of strategies are yours alone.

Getting on with Life Blueprint

MONTH	Long-term PMS Plan
POST MENSTRUAL WEEKS	▪ STOP PMS formula. SWITCH BACK to daily multiple vitamin-mineral supplement (with juice + breakfast). Take 1,000 mg. of calcium with dinner or at bedtime with juice. **Diet:** **Exercise:** **Relaxation:** **Thought-Changing:** **Time Management:** **Relationships:** **Alternative Therapies:** **Other** (medications, counseling, other personal strategies):
PRE MENSTRUAL WEEKS	▪ STOP regular multivitamin-mineral supplement; START PMS Formula vitamin-mineral supplement. Continue taking calcium supplement. **Diet:** **Exercise:** **Relaxation:** **Thought-Changing:** **Time Management:** **Relationships:** **Alternative Therapies:** **Other** (medications, counseling, other personal strategies):

Use the first day of your period as a time to have an appointment with yourself. You'll need to begin a new "PMS Tracking Chart" anyway so use this natural pause as an opportunity to focus on yourself, celebrate what you've accomplished in the last month, and embrace the challenges that lie ahead. Indeed, this is an ideal time to think about what you want to change about your life in the coming month. Do you want to create or join a support group or take a meditation or yoga class to hone your relaxation skills? Would it help to plan exercise sessions for first thing in the morning before countless excuses or obstacles stand in your way? Would you like to schedule a particular project for a time of the month when you can tap your natural, cyclical surge in creativity? By coordinating your activities with your menstrual cycle, you'll not only be managing your PMS but learning to live in sync with your body's natural rhythms.

■ *What If . . . ?* ■

Even the best-laid plans don't always have the effect we want them to. Based on real-life situations that were encountered by women in my PMS studies, this section offers suggestions on what to do if you encounter some of the more common problems that can arise as you implement or modify your PMS plan.

■ *What should I do if I don't do what I planned to do?*

If you didn't get started because you planned too many strategies and wound up feeling overwhelmed, pare down your list. Plan smaller, more manageable activities or plot them for shorter periods of time. Or do a time-analysis of your current activities to figure out how and when you can fit your chosen activities into your schedule. It's also possible that you need to ask for help—from an exercise buddy, your spouse, a friend, or a support group. Sometimes talking through the logistics can make a big difference.

■ *What if my symptoms aren't decreasing in severity?*

Pull out your PMS Tracking Charts and clarify which symptoms are not decreasing in severity and whether there is a pattern. If you have one or two physical symptoms that didn't change in spite of implementing your plan, try out the remedies in the "Symptom-Solution Section" in this chapter. If you are experiencing ongoing worry, mood swings, obsessions, depression, or persistent fatigue, especially in the postmenstrual phase, page ahead to Chapter Thirteen; you may need further evaluation by a health professional. If, however, you are virtually free of symptoms in the postmenstrual phase but some of the premenstrual turmoil and blues symptoms remain (albeit at a lower intensity), check out Chapters Eleven and Twelve for additional measures that may help.

- *What if my PMS comes back after a hiatus even though I'm doing every-thing in my plan?*

Sometimes women need to reassess their symptoms and their PMS plan from the beginning. It may be that you have some new symptoms or that your menstrual cycle is becoming irregular as you move into the peri-menopausal transition. Or maybe you've stopped doing some part of your PMS plan and you need to "restart" your treatment program. It's possible that some bad habits may have slipped into your routine without your even realizing it. Just go back to Chapter Three, reassess your PMS symptoms, and begin tracking anew. Keeping your own "PMS Notebook," which you read about in Chapter Three, will allow you to compare your experiences from different time periods.

- *What if my premenstrual symptoms vary considerably from month to month?*

It is not uncommon for either the number of symptoms or the severity of symptoms to change from one cycle to another. One month you might have more physical discomfort and fewer mood symptoms, for example, while the next month you could have the reverse pattern. If this every-other-month pattern is consistent, then you will need to adapt your PMS plan accordingly. In other words, every other month, you will want to start taking NSAIDs as soon as you feel or see your period starting if you often experience menstrual cramps or headaches. But remember that regular aerobic exercise will likely go a long way toward decreasing these pain symptoms. In the months when your mood symptoms are more severe, you will want to do more relaxation and cognitive stress-management strategies.

- *What if my PMS improves but I continue to feel tired for most of the month?*

Fatigue is a common symptom that's associated with many different health problems as well as stress. In fact, it's one of the most common rea-sons people seek medical care. If you have tried the various diet, nutritional supplement, and exercise strategies, and your fatigue has diminished some-what but continues even after the end of your period, then you may have an underlying medical or psychiatric condition that needs further evaluation. See Chapter Thirteen for more information about conditions that are exacerbated by the menstrual cycle.

- *What if my symptoms go away?*

First, get down on your knees and bow to the goddess of PMS relief. But don't stop your PMS plan! Obviously, it has worked. Why mess with success? Besides, your premenstrual symptoms could make a comeback at some point, perhaps as you enter the perimenopausal transition or after you have a baby. In the meantime, your personalized PMS plan is also a package of strategies that can be the basis for lifelong health-enhancement.

- *What if I want to get pregnant?*

For some women, pregnancy is a cure for PMS, while for others, their symptoms worsen in the first trimester. If you are simply contemplating a pregnancy, you can continue with your cyclical vitamin and mineral supplements until you stop using contraception. Once you are actively trying to conceive, you should take only your regular multivitamin and mineral supplement, not the PMS-formula supplement. And if you're using herbal remedies, a prescription drug, or OTC medications, consult your doctor or midwife to make sure it's safe to continue. Otherwise, you can safely continue all the other PMS plan strategies.

- *What if my mood symptoms persist or worsen?*

If you find that your premenstrual "Turmoil" or "Blues" symptoms decrease in severity but remain in the mild-to-moderate intensity or increase during the winter months, you may want to add other strategies to your PMS plan. Herbal therapies such as Kava Kava or St. John's Wort or light therapy for winter depression may be helpful additions to your plan. See Chapter Eleven for alternative therapies. But if you notice anxiety or panicky feelings that do not respond to interventions, persist all month long, or become debilitating, you may have a panic disorder. In that case, see your health-care provider or a qualified mental health professional. Similarly, if your depressive symptoms become increasingly intense or you have persistent thoughts of harming yourself, see a health professional or a local crisis center.

PART THREE

The Next Step

11

Emerging Therapies for PMS

I f you haven't found sufficient relief with the preceding strategies, you may want to consider trying one or more of the following newer techniques. Several promising alternative or complementary therapies for PMS have come to light in recent years. These approaches are different from those used by conventional, Western medical practitioners, and while the science behind many of these nonmedicinal remedies is sparse, many of these treatments do have some research to support their use (in addition to a couple thousand years of empirical evidence, in some cases). We've included them because alternative or complementary treatments such as herbal remedies, homeopathy, massage, and nutritional supplements are quite popular among women who have PMS.

While the use of light therapy sprang from high-tech research interventions, many of the therapies included here—such as acupuncture—are based on centuries-old practices or ancient healing systems. Indeed, many of these techniques are based on Eastern philosophies, which do not separate the body from the mind, or health from lifestyle. Instead, the view is of a woman's body as an integrated whole, with body and mind working in concert. The aim behind these disciplines is to create balance and harmony in the body, to produce subtle effects over time, or to bolster the body's own healing abilities rather than relying on a potent drug that would intervene in a more aggressive way. In other words, they're trying to help the body heal itself from the inside out rather than trying to fix the body from the outside.

Because of the complexity of these various approaches, we can't possibly do them justice. What we have strived to do is to give you an overview of how they could help relieve various premenstrual symptoms. Keep in mind: To err on the side of caution, we have included herbal or nutritional remedies only if they are considered safe and have well-documented efficacy studies behind them.

Acupuncture:

In traditional Chinese medicine, both herbs and acupuncture are used separately or in combination to treat health conditions that result from disruptions to the flow of the body's vital energy (qi or chi), an imbalance between the eternal opposites of yin and yang. Acupuncture, the ancient Chinese art of needle placement, has been found to be helpful in the treatment of severe PMS. Recently, some doctors and nurses have become licensed acupuncturists and use the technique as part of their conventional medical practice. Considered a form of energy medicine, acupuncture treatment manipulates the vital energy sources of the body by introducing ultra-thin needles to specific points along the "meridians," the energy pathways, of the body. Recent studies from the National Institutes of Health have found acupuncture to be effective for pain syndromes such as headaches and low back pain. If premenstrual or menstrual cramps, low back pain, joint pain or headaches persist, acupuncture may be an effective alternative therapy. Look for a licensed practitioner of Chinese medicine or acupuncture. Licensing requirements vary by state but many rely on certification by the National Certification Commission for Acupuncture and Oriental Medicine as part of their licensure requirements.

The Healing Touch:

On the scale of feel-good treatments, massage ranks way up there. But it also has therapeutic benefits. Stroking and kneading the body's skin and muscle tissue has been found to relieve physical and emotional tension, increase circulation, improve sleep, enhance immune function, and promote feelings of well-being. What's more, a study of 35 PMS sufferers, published in *Obstetrics and Gynecology*, found that reflexology—applying manual pressure to specific points on the hands or feet—significantly decreased their symptoms. While there are many different types of massage, the two most widely available forms are Swedish massage and Oriental massage (including reflexology, shiatsu, and acupressure). Massage therapists often specialize in one or more types of massage with sessions lasting 30 to 90 minutes. You can also learn some massage techniques to use on yourself or you can teach a friend or partner some massage basics.

Acupressure combines the benefits of massage with the therapeutic aspects of acupuncture. Not only can it be used as a form of self-care for the symptoms already described, but it can also be an effective treatment for acute and chronic pain including cyclical pelvic pain. While delicately puncturing the skin with a needle is the usual method of stimulating specific anatomic points in the body for therapeutic purposes, as is done with acupuncture, acupressure is an alternative method that involves applying direct physical pressure to energy points and channels that are used in acupuncture. In a recent clinical trial I conducted with women who had moderate to severe menstrual pain, an acupressure device in the form of an underpant-like garment provided clinically significant symptom relief. Women using the acupressure device also used less pain medication than women in the control group. You can learn different ways of applying pressure that can relieve emotional tension and physical discomfort from various self-help manuals. (See the Resources guide in the Appendix for suggestions.)

Chiropractic:
Although therapeutic manipulation of the body was a component of medicine for thousands of years, only two forms remain as part of modern medicine—chiropractic and osteopathy. (*Chiropractic* means "done by hand" in Greek.) Research has demonstrated that chiropractic treatments are beneficial for back pain, significantly reducing pain and suffering as well as functional limitations. In studies of migraine headaches and menstrual cramps, chiropractic adjustment was more effective than the placebo treatment. And a recent randomized, placebo-controlled study of chiropractic adjustment (a.k.a., spinal manipulation) in 25 women with PMS confirmed that chiropractic

therapy can reduce symptoms in some women with PMS. The theory is that spinal manipulation may reduce the production of prostaglandins and help re-balance ovarian hormones.

Homeopathy:
This is a holistic treatment system that's based on the principle that giving a person the right dose of a natural substance that might disturb the body in the wrong amounts can actually trigger healing. Homeopathic remedies were first developed by an eighteenth-century physician named Samuel Hahnemann, who focused on healing the whole person, not just her symptoms. Evidence that the more than 1,000 homeopathic remedies—such as those extracted from plants, minerals, and animal products—work is primarily anecdotal, and many mainstream researchers reject homeopathic theories of action. In a meta-analysis of 105 clinical trials of homeopathic treatments, however, the researchers found that 75 percent of interpretable trials showed a positive result. More recently, a randomized, controlled, double-blind clinical trial at The Hebrew University, Hadassah Medical School, in Israel found that 90 percent of the women experienced an improvement of more than 30 percent in their premenstrual symptoms after an oral dose of a homeopathic medication. While homeopathic remedies have no side effects and are available without a prescription, it is wise to consult a professional homeopath who can help you choose the most appropriate treatments, especially if your symptoms are severe and haven't responded to other treatments.

Light Therapy:
There's no question that the menstrual cycle—as well as its related hormones in the brain and ovaries—is influenced by natural light. And research indicates that sunlight increases the level of the feel-good brain chemical serotonin for some people. What's more, studies by Barbara Parry, M.D., a psychiatrist at the University of California, San Diego, suggest a link between PMS and Seasonal Affective Disorder (SAD), a type of depression that typically occurs in the fall and winter months when levels of natural light decline in most areas of the country. In women who are highly sensitive to light, exposure to full-spectrum light, including ultraviolet light, has been found to decrease

the mood and depressive symptoms of PMS. In a recent study at the University of British Columbia in Vancouver, researchers found that women with severe PMS who were treated with 30 minutes of evening light therapy for two weeks during the luteal phase of their menstrual cycles experienced a significant reduction in depression and premenstrual tension.

For women who feel depressed all month long during the fall and winter months and experience an increased severity of premenstrual mood symptoms during these seasons, light therapy may be considered a viable option. One theory is that bright light corrects disturbances in the body's internal sleep-wake cycle that are linked with PMS; or, it could be that the light promotes the effects of the feel-good brain chemical serotonin. If you're interested in light therapy, the first step should be to consult a psychotherapist or mental health counselor.

If you aren't interested in undergoing formal light therapy but you would like to brighten your world at certain times of the month, that's an option, too. Keep in mind: Recent research suggests that exposure to morning light may be especially beneficial for women with PMS so you may want to time your exposure accordingly. Some suggestions for increasing light exposure:

- Exercise outside whenever possible; even cloudy days give more full-spectrum light than indoor light.

- Use full spectrum lights—either incandescent or fluorescent—in your home or office whenever possible. The recommended range for the amount of light is from 2,500 to 10,000 lux (a measure of light intensity).

- Switch to full-spectrum UV-transmitting eyeglasses or contacts for at least a portion of the day since most sunglasses and many prescription lenses block ultraviolet (UV) light.

- Move your desk or work space close to a natural light source if you spend many hours indoors. If that isn't possible, get up every hour or so and walk over to a bright window.

- If at all possible, avoid shift-work or working nights as this can disrupt your sleep patterns and increase PMS severity.

- Try a full-spectrum light box. These commercially available devices generally run $150 to $500 but may be covered by your health insurance plan if a health-care provider prescribes the device.

Whether or not you want to explore one of these emerging therapies is up to you. But if you feel as though you've exhausted the options in your PMS plan and you're in search of further nonpharmaceutical relief, you may want to consider one of these healing systems. Before embarking on any new therapy, we encourage you to educate yourself about the promises and pitfalls of these treatments, just as you would before taking a medication or electing to undergo a surgical procedure. To help you get started, you'll find a number of books, organizations, and websites listed in the Resources section of the Appendix.

The Herbal Medicine Cabinet

Plants—their leaves, roots, seeds, bark, fruit, and stems—have been used for centuries as medicines, and herbs are still a primary treatment for health conditions in many countries throughout the world. Herbal medicines may be gentler than their pharmaceutical relatives but their active ingredients can have profound effects. While approximately 600 botanical remedies are sold in the U.S., the Food and Drug Administration (FDA) lists nine herbs that can cause serious health problems; these include chaparral, comfrey, germander, jin bu huan, lobelia, magnolia, ma huang (or ephedra), stephania, and yohimbe. Of course, this does not mean that the remaining 591 are safe and effective. The herbal terrain is still a bit like the wild, wild west—uncharted territory, scientifically speaking. Not only are herbs unregulated by the FDA—in terms of safety, efficacy, strength, or purity—but there is a lack of sufficient clinical trials on the benefits and side effects of herbs, which makes it difficult to recommend safe and effective herbal preparations. Using herbs can also be challenging because the amount of active ingredients in one dose can vary widely among different brands of the same herb. Or, an herb may be available as an extract in a capsule, in a tablet or as a tea, making it difficult to gauge your dosage.

With all that being said, several herbs do seem to have beneficial effects on PMS, as well as depression, anxiety, insomnia, and memory problems. In addition, psychotherapeutic herbs such as St. John's Wort have been found to be effective for major depression and could be used for severe premenstrual depression. And Kava Kava, a root from the South Pacific, has been used as a natural remedy for anxiety symptoms and may help with serious premenstrual jitters. All of these herbs are available without a prescription at pharmacies and health-food stores. Because not all herbs have enough clinical or research evidence to say with certainty that they are safe and effective, only those herbs that have been recommended by the German Commission E—basically, the equivalent of an FDA for herbs, this organization was established more than 20 years ago and has reviewed all the available literature on more than 300 herbs—or by the late Varro Tyler, Ph.D., a professor of pharmacognosy at Purdue University and author of *The Honest Herbal*, are included here. To learn about safe, therapeutic dosages, you may want to consult *The American Pharmaceutical Association Practical Guide to Natural Medicines*. (For further resources, see the Appendix.)

VITEX AGNUS-CASTUS (CHASTE TREE BERRY)

Native to valleys and riverbanks of the Mediterranean and central Asia, chaste tree (also called Vitex) is a shrub that produces dark brown to black fruit the size of a peppercorn. Preparations of the fruit—as an extract or in powdered form—have been approved by German health authorities for the treatment of menstrual irregularities, such as PMS and breast pain that's associated with a woman's period. Thanks to its dopamine-like activity and effect on the pituitary gland, chaste tree berry extracts help to reinstate the normal balance between estrogen and progesterone during the luteal phase of the menstrual cycle. Clinical trials have shown that chaste tree berry extract keeps the overproduction of progesterone in check and effectively reduces breast pain that's associated with a woman's period.

In the first placebo-controlled trial to clearly demonstrate the herb's effectiveness in treating PMS, German scientists found that women taking 20 mg. of Vitex reported a 52 percent overall reduction in PMS symptoms compared with only 24 percent for those taking a placebo. Only 5 percent of the women who took Vitex experienced mild side effects such as acne, skin rash, and bleeding between their periods; none of these symptoms caused women to drop out of the study.

Although chaste tree berry extracts do not contain hormones, they should not be used with birth control pills or other hormone replacement therapies without the guidance of a health-care professional. Chaste tree berry extract also should not be used during pregnancy as it can stimulate premature lactation.

EVENING PRIMROSE OIL

The seed oil of the evening primrose, a weed that is native to North America, is high in the essential fatty acid gamma linolenic acid (or GLA), which is a precursor to prostaglandin. Over 120 studies in 15 countries have reported on the potential use of evening primrose oil and the studies of its use for PMS suggest that it helps to regulate hormones. Although the results of research have been mixed, some researchers have found that consuming evening primrose oil supplements decreases premenstrual mood symptoms, breast pain, and fluid retention. Safety of the herb seems well established but about 2 percent of those who take evening primrose oil may experience stomach discomfort, nausea, or headache.

CHAMOMILE

A plant that's a member of the daisy family, chamomile has been studied extensively in Europe and is used primarily as a digestive aid, an anti-inflammatory for skin conditions, an antispasmodic for menstrual cramps, and a mild sedative and sleep aid. The flower heads are safe enough to use with children and during pregnancy in tea form. Be careful with this one, though, if you have other allergic conditions, particularly hay fever: The herb contains varying amounts of allergens as well as pollen so it could elicit a reaction in those who have allergies.

FEVERFEW

An aromatic, perennial herb, feverfew has been used to treat headaches, stomachaches, menstrual cramps, arthritis, and fevers. Clinical trials of the herb feverfew demonstrate effectiveness for relieving and preventing migraine headaches as well as the nausea and vomiting that often accompany these debilitating headaches. Results from a crossover, placebo-controlled trial found that those who were treated with dried feverfew leaves experienced fewer migraines, less severe attacks, and less vomiting than those in the control group did. It is available in many forms, including as an extract, tea, and capsules. Although few problems have been reported regarding feverfew, its long-term safety has not been established. (You may want to steer clear of this herb if you are allergic to ragweed.)

GINKGO BILOBA

Chinese healers have been using the leaves of the ginkgo tree since ancient times because of their medicinal properties. The use of ginkgo has greatly increased in Europe and America since 1994, when German health authorities approved a standardized form of the leaf extract for the treatment of dementia. Research has found that ginkgo leaf extracts may improve memory and learning, enhance blood flow, and have neuroprotective and anti-anxiety effects, as well as interfering with the factor that activates blood clotting. Ginkgo may be beneficial through its action both as a blood-thinner—thereby promoting increased circulation in the brain and the extremities—and as an antioxidant—helping to deactivate the free radicals that can cause cellular damage.

In humans, side effects are rare and the toxicity of ginkgo leaf extracts is very low. In a German post-marketing surveillance study of nearly 11,000 people who were treated with ginkgo, only 183 reported side effects such as nausea, diarrhea, and headache. In addition, there have been a few reports of bleeding problems that were associated with ginkgo treatment. Ginkgo comes in tablets, capsules, concentrated drops, tinctures, and extracts.

Psychotherapeutic Herbs

Specific herbs, prescribed in pharmacological doses, have been used to treat severe premenstrual depression and anxiety-type symptoms. Hypericum, or St. John's Wort, has been found to be effective for major depression and could be used for severe premenstrual depression as well. Kava Kava, a root from the South Pacific, has been used as a natural remedy for anxiety symptoms. These herbs are available over the counter at pharmacies and health-food stores and can be tried before using the stronger antidepressant medications. Results may be noticeable immediately for some herbs like Kava Kava but it could take weeks for others to show effects.

There are many relaxant and sedative herbs that work for both simple anxiety and insomnia, but these should only be used for a brief time along with other nonpharmacological methods. Using these for a few days when your PMS turmoil symptoms are at their highest or during times of high stress—before exams or a difficult meeting, or after a traumatic event, for example—is fine but don't make a habit of it. If anxiety or insomnia become a chronic problem, page ahead to Chapter Thirteen and consider consulting a health professional who has experience with anxiety and/or sleep disorders.

VALERIAN

The name sounds like the anti-anxiety drug Valium but valerian is a perennial herb with white or reddish flowers. In Europe, it is a popular botanical medicine that is used for its mild sedative and calming properties, even though it has an unpleasant odor. German health authorities have indicated that valerian is an effective treatment for "restlessness and nervous disturbance of sleep." Valerian is a popular sleep remedy but has had few confirmatory studies; however, a recent German study found that after one month of treatment valerian was a better sleep inducer than the placebo. In all of the studies, most patients described the medication as extremely helpful. No side effects have been reported, and most participants said they would purchase this product themselves if their insomnia continued or recurred. In humans, valerian seems to be quite safe but it may cause mild, temporary stomach upset. It is not addictive nor does it have any "hangover" effects like synthetic sedatives do. (Just be sure to avoid using it with other sedatives, antidepressants, or tranquilizers.)

KAVA KAVA

A South Pacific root and a psychoactive member of the pepper family, Kava Kava (or just simply kava) has long been used for short-term relief from stress and anxiety. Several placebo-controlled trials have shown significant anti-anxiety effects from the use of kava. It can also help with insomnia. In contrast to the benzodiazepine sedatives and tricyclic antidepressants, both of which are used to treat anxiety disorders, treatment with kava does not lead to a loss of response to the herb over time.

Even though it has a long tradition as a treatment for "states of nervous anxiety, tension, and agitation," recent reports of liver problems have called kava's safety into question. The majority of these adverse effects took place in people who were taking kava in combination with prescription drugs. In January 2002, France banned its sale, Switzerland pulled it off the market, and Britain asked for manufacturers to voluntarily withdraw kava from the market. In the meantime, the FDA is investigating whether kava's use in dietary supplements poses a risk to public health.

Until more is known, make sure you don't exceed the recommended dosage of kava or take it for more than four weeks. (You can stay abreast of the latest news on kava by checking some of the websites listed in the Resources section.) Therapeutic doses may result in mild gastrointestinal complaints or allergic skin reactions but these occur in only about 2 percent of people who try them. To avoid dangerous interactions, kava should not be used with alcohol; nor should it be combined with other anti-anxiety medications. It should not be used by women during pregnancy or by people with depression or known liver problems.

ST. JOHN'S WORT

St. John's Wort is a common perennial plant that has gained much popularity in the United States as a treatment for mild to moderate depression. In a recent meta-analysis of German studies, St. John's Wort outdid the placebo for mild-to-moderate depression and had fewer side effects than antidepressant drugs: In fact, 55 percent of those receiving the herb improved, compared with 22 percent of those receiving a placebo. The exact mechanism of its action is unknown but it is thought to act like SSRI antidepressants, fooling the brain into thinking that more serotonin is present than actually is there. This tends to elevate mood and provide emotional stability. Unlike antidepressant drugs, however, St. John's Wort doesn't cause drowsiness or interact in an adverse fashion with alcohol. Although it has an excellent safety record, more information is needed on its efficacy compared with SSRIs since it has only been compared with the older tricyclic antidepressants.

With St. John's Wort, side effects are generally mild and include gastrointestinal symptoms and fatigue but these affect only 2 to 3 percent of people who take it. The most predictable effect seems to be photosensitization—an increased sensitivity of the skin to sunlight—especially in fair-skinned people if the herb is taken at high doses; fortunately, this effect is usually transient and disappears within a few days of discontinuing the drug. To date, no effects on fertility or reproduction have been found with St. John's Wort. In April 2000, the FDA issued an advisory cautioning that when St. John's Wort is taken with any of the following drugs, effectiveness of the medication may be reduced: Cardiac drugs, antidepressants, oral contraceptives, antiseizure drugs, anti-cancer drugs, and transplant anti-rejection drugs.

PASSION FLOWER

Passion flower may not be recognized as an effective agent in the U.S., but it is included in many preparations, often in combination with other herbs that are sold in Europe as mild sedatives. It has been recommended for the treatment of dysmenorrhea, PMS, and general nervousness. Although it appears to be safe, no clinical trials have been conducted to examine its use as a single agent. No adverse reactions have been reported, other than one unconvincing case of hypersensitivity vasculitis (inflammation of the blood vessels, in simpler terms).

◼ *Guidelines for Using Herbs* ◼

Although most dietary supplements that are available in retail stores may seem safe, they are not risk-free. One potential problem is that people often mix herbs or dietary supplements with drugs. That could be a big mistake. Here are several savvy guidelines about how to use herbs safely:

- Always inform your primary-care health provider of any drugs you're using, including herbal remedies, especially if you have an underlying medical problem (such as heart disease) or a chronic health condition (such as asthma).

- Stop taking the herb immediately if you experience side effects. Notify your primary-care provider of your experience.
- Do not take herbs if you are pregnant or nursing, unless it's under the advice of your doctor or midwife.
- Select herbal products carefully. Purchase only those that list the herb's common and scientific names, the name and address of the manufacturer, a batch or lot number, an expiration date, dosing guidelines, potential side effects, and details of how quality is ensured.

Nutritional Supplements

With mounting scientific evidence on how sound dietary practices can contribute to health and healing, growing attention is being paid to the mechanisms that may be responsible for those therapeutic effects. Nevertheless, there is still a scarcity of research on some of the newer nutritional remedies such as the use of amino acids, essential fatty acids, and other neuroactive substances, such as SAM-e.

AMINO ACID SUPPLEMENTS

Amino acids are building blocks of protein structures in the body such as the skin, hair, bones, muscles, and hormones. About half of the amino acids that are important for human metabolism are not made in the body and must be obtained by eating protein or by taking supplements. When taken in large doses, amino acids have drug-like effects and should be treated with the same caution that you would exercise when taking any prescription medication or herbal remedy.

As far as PMS is concerned, a few amino acids are necessary for the production of certain brain neurotransmitters that are related to mood. Tyrosine, L-tryptophan, and gamma aminobutyric acid (GABA) are influential in the pathophysiology of depression and anxiety, for example. But while research has demonstrated the safety and effectiveness of GABA and recent studies of phenylalanine and tyrosine show promising results, until there are more complete efficacy studies, it is too early to recommend amino acid supplements as potential therapies for PMS. Although there have been no adverse effects reported for either tyrosine or carnitine, the deaths that were associated in 1989 with contaminated L-tryptophan supplements are a potent reminder that these supplements are not always benign dietary aids.

Fortunately, there's an alternative to using amino acid supplements—and that is to increase your intake of food sources that are high in these amino acids. You'll find a list of foods that are high in tyrosine and tryptophan in Chapter Four.

OMEGA-3 ESSENTIAL FATTY ACIDS

New research suggests that in addition to decreasing cardiovascular risk factors and cyclical pelvic pain, omega-3 fatty acids show promise for the treatment of depression. In one study, people with bipolar disorder who were given dietary supplements with the two fatty acids in the omega-3s, DHA (docosahexaenoic acid) and EPA (eicosapentaenoic acid), showed marked mood stabilization. It has been theorized that consuming adequate amounts of polyunsaturated fatty acids, particularly DHA, may reduce the development of depression just as they also reduce the risk of coronary artery disease. In addition, omega-3 fatty acids have been found to relieve menstrual pain. Other research has found that people with rheumatoid arthritis and irritable bowel symptoms were able to use less NSAID medications if they consumed omega-3 fatty acids.

With high doses of fish oil—such as those that were used in the depression research—some people may experience nausea, loose stools, and "fishy" breath. These side effects have not been found in studies that have used lower but still therapeutic levels for other conditions. Omega-3 fatty acids are safe to use during pregnancy and lactation. Of course, eating fish is the best way to get omega-3 fatty acids. To increase your intake of these fatty acids from your diet, aim to eat fatty fish such as bluefish, herring, mackerel, salmon, sardines, or tuna twice a week. If you want to try fish oil supplements, look for a commercial preparation that contains 1,000 mg. of EPA and 700 mg. of DHA—and take it daily in one or two divided doses for two months. To maximize absorption, make sure that your daily multivitamin and mineral supplement also includes vitamin E or take 400 IU of vitamin E daily.

SAM-E

It's not a drug; it's not an herb. S-adenosylmethionine, or SAM-e, is a mouthful of a name for a molecule that is manufactured in the body from the amino acid methionine during metabolism. Available for years in Europe, SAM-e has been shown to be both safe and effective in treating depression—comparable to that of standard tricyclic antidepressants, according to a 1994 meta-analysis. Teodoro Bottiglieri, Ph.D., a neuropharmacologist at the Baylor University Medical Center's Institute of Metabolic Disease in Dallas, Texas, has been studying SAM-e for more than 15 years and considers it to be safe and effective for mild to moderate depressive symptoms. (If you have a bipolar disorder, however, SAM-e can induce mania.) It has also been found to be helpful in reducing joint pain that's associated with osteoarthritis, and it's a useful alternative for people who experience unpleasant side effects with NSAIDs. As for its own side effects, these are minimal; however, in about 2 to 3 percent of people, SAM-e has been reported to cause transient insomnia, mild nervousness, and a lack of appetite.

Unfortunately, there is no way to find a standardized dose of SAM-e. And because raw SAM-e degrades quickly unless it is stored at a proper temperature, there is no guarantee that the pills you buy will retain their potency since there's no way to know if they have been properly handled. The other drawback: SAM-e is very expensive. A daily dose can range from $2.50 to $18, and you need to take it over a few weeks to see results.

Medicating Measures

Truth be told, the natural route isn't always the best way to go for women with very serious PMS symptoms. After all, some women experience severe PMS, noncyclical mood disorders, seasonal depression, or intense menstrual pain that may benefit from medication in combination with various aspects of a PMS symptom management program. Others may be so acutely sensitive to hormonal fluctuations that it may make sense to suppress these swings for peace of mind and body.

For those women who find that they have symptoms such as depression or anxiety all month long but that their symptoms tend to worsen during the premenstrual phase, it's a good idea to discuss this with your health-care practitioner. Certain hormonal therapies, antidepressants, anti-anxiety agents, and forms of counseling have been found to be particularly helpful in dealing with some of these moods. In addition, oral contraceptives have been found to be effective for relief of menstrual discomfort such as intense cramps and menstrual migraines, while diuretics are often prescribed for some of the physical symptoms such as severe premenstrual fluid retention and weight gain.

At this point, you are probably reading this section because you have one or more symptoms that have continued to be severe in spite of everything you've been doing with your PMS solution. Many women say they would prefer not to take medications. But if you have tried all of the other strategies and you are still experiencing bothersome premenstrual symptoms, you might want to consider combining drug therapies with your PMS management strategies. In this chapter, we'll review the most commonly used medications for PMS-related woes and those that have the most evidence for safety and effectiveness. Keep in mind, however, that most medications have some side effects; we have alerted you to these as well. Since most medications that would be useful for PMS require a prescription, you'll need to consult your health-care provider before using most of these pharmacological therapies.

Antidepressants:

At first blush, using an antidepressant to treat PMS may seem like overkill. But researchers now know that there is a reduction in the mood-enhancing brain chemical serotonin prior to menstruation, which may contribute to premenstrual mood swings. A class of antidepressant medications called selective serotonin reuptake inhibitors (SSRIs, for short) increases levels of serotonin in the brain, thereby effectively treating noncyclical depression as well as the severe mood symptoms of PMS. Some of the common brand names are Prozac (fluoxetine), Zoloft (sertraline), and Paxil (paroxetine). Recently, a new form of fluoxetine was approved by the FDA for the treatment of PMDD (premenstrual dysphoric disorder) or severe PMS under the brand name Sarafem.

These medications can often help with the more severe mood symptoms of PMS—and a woman doesn't necessarily have to take them all month long to benefit. Taking one of these antidepressants during the luteal phase—the second half of the menstrual cycle—is often sufficient for many women. Or, a woman may be able to get by with a lower dose if she's using it in combination with her personalized PMS plan.

While clinical studies of SSRIs for depression and obsessive-compulsive disorders have found that efficacy is reached only after four to eight weeks of daily use, it appears that in some cases of severe PMS SSRIs may become effective within a few days and, in most cases, within one menstrual cycle. The theory is that this effect may reflect

SSRI action at a different receptor site from that in affective disorders, such as clinical depression. The rapid onset of action in severe PMS allows intermittent dosing regimens to induce a temporary increase in serotonin concentrations during the luteal phase, when a woman with PMS needs this most. In a recent meta-analysis of 15 randomized, placebo-controlled trials, there was no difference between the intermittent and continuous dosing regimen in the treatment of PMS. Despite such encouraging news, it's important to remember that antidepressants aren't a panacea for PMS: Research has found that 40 percent of women with PMS don't respond to Prozac or other SSRIs.

Moreover, these antidepressants are not without side effects. The most common side effects are headaches, sleep disturbances, dizziness, dry mouth, and decreased libido. Other, less often reported side effects include decreased appetite, weight loss, drowsiness, impaired concentration, altered taste, nausea, diarrhea, and nervousness. If these occur, they can usually be lessened with lower dosages of the medications.

Anti-anxiety drugs:

For years, anti-anxiety medications or tranquilizers have been used for anxiety symptoms that are severe or noncyclical. These medications are also used with psychotherapy for the treatment of panic attacks. The most commonly prescribed anti-anxiety medication is alprazolam (Xanax). Other tranquilizers include diazepam (Valium), lorazepam (Ativan), and buspirone (BuSpar).

Research on the use of anti-anxiety medications has generally shown mixed results. In the only randomized, crossover, placebo-controlled clinical trial of alprazolam for use during the premenstrual phase, women taking the drug experienced less anxiety, depression, and headache. The bad news is, side effects such as drowsiness and sedation and medication tolerance (loss of a normal response to the drug) caused high dropout rates in this trial. Alprazolam has also been shown to increase food intake premenstrually, which could make it hard to control food cravings or binges if you're vulnerable to these.

These medications are for short-term use only—continued use should not exceed eight weeks without medical evaluation—because physical and psychological dependencies can occur quickly with these drugs. The body builds up a tolerance so you end up needing a higher dose to get the same effects over time. The other risk is that if you rely on these instead of developing good stress management practices, you may feel the need to pop a pill every time something upsetting happens. In other words, it's easy to become addicted to these drugs, physically and emotionally.

Even in the short-term, side effects can include visual problems, mood swings, and joint stiffness. Other, less frequently reported side effects include drowsiness, headache, dizziness, blurred vision, dry mouth, weakness, confusion, nausea, constipation, agitation, and depression. Oral contraceptives can increase the potency of anti-anxiety drugs, which can increase the risk of side effects. By contrast, alcohol, if consumed while taking an anti-anxiety drug, increases depression of the central nervous system, which could make you excessively drowsy and slow your breathing down to the point where you may not be getting enough oxygen.

Sleeping aids:

Prescription sleep aids are part of the family of sedative-hypnotic medications that include anti-anxiety agents. Drugs such as Ambien, Halcion, and Restoril will initially improve sleep problems by inducing and maintaining sleep but they lose their effectiveness quickly and often cause more sleep problems by disrupting the normal stages of sleep. What's more, these medications can act like "memory robbers," causing forgetfulness, mental fogginess, and impaired concentration. With the short-acting sleep medications, such as Halcion, some women experience a rebound anxiety when the drug wears off. For these reasons, among others, some doctors recommend low doses of some of the older sedating antidepressants that boost serotonin—drugs like trazodone (Desyrel), amitriptyline (Elavil), or imipramine (Tofranil)—as well as the newer SSRI antidepressants as treatment for insomnia.

Diuretics:

A class of drugs called diuretics is often prescribed to reduce premenstrual fluid retention—such as abdominal bloating and swelling of the hands, legs, ankles, and feet—and may also decrease headaches that are associated with these premenstrual fluid shifts. The downside is these drugs can deplete potassium levels in the body and create an electrolyte imbalance, which would result in further stimulation of the autonomic nervous system. When this happens, weakness, fatigue, dizziness, lightheadedness, nausea, muscle cramping, and sweating can occur. The risk of potassium depletion is higher with the more potent thiazide diuretics but it can also happen with herbal diuretics. To prevent potassium depletion, potassium supplements are often recommended with the use of diuretics along with dietary forms of potassium (bananas, potatoes, cantaloupe, apricots, lentils, and so on).

Another type of diuretic that creates a more gradual loss of fluid and is potassium-sparing is spironolactone. This is a better alternative to the stronger thiazide diuretics but it can also produce side effects such as headaches, skin itching, nausea, and diarrhea. Since you could be trading one set of unpleasant symptoms for another with the use of diuretics, you may be better off sticking with the diet and lifestyle alterations (from Chapter Ten) unless your health-care practitioner specifically recommends one of these drugs.

Prostaglandin inhibitors:
Since prostaglandins are known to play a role in stimulating uterine cramping and bleeding during menstruation, drugs that inhibit the production of these agents are often used to relieve the pain-related symptoms of PMS. The primary class of prostaglandin inhibitors are nonsteroidal anti-inflammatory drugs (NSAIDs), which include ibuprofen, naproxen, ketoprofen, and mefenamic acid. These are available in over-the-counter forms (such as Advil, Motrin, Nuprin, and Aleve) and prescription forms (including Anaprox, Orudis, Ponstel, and stronger doses of Motrin). If taken at the appropriate dosages (see Chapter Ten's "Symptom-Solution Section" for recommendations), they will decrease premenstrual pelvic cramping as well as backaches, body aches and pains, and perhaps fluid retention since these drugs act on the smooth muscles of the uterus, abdomen, and intestines. Side effects include gastrointestinal discomfort, commonly in the form of pain, nausea, heartburn, or indigestion, but this discomfort can be minimized by consuming food with the medication.

HORMONAL TREATMENTS

It may sound counterintuitive to treat a condition such as PMS, which is related to hormonal fluctuations, with more hormones but it can make a substantial difference for some women with severe PMS. To date, two forms of hormonal treatment have been shown to reduce severe premenstrual symptoms. One provides supplementation with natural forms of progesterone. The other suppresses ovulation using oral contraceptives.

Progesterone Therapy:

Natural progesterone is a hormone that is produced by the ovaries and the adrenal glands. It is secreted into the bloodstream where it circulates throughout the body and stimulates receptors in the breast, uterus, brain, central nervous system, as well as the cardiovascular and musculoskeletal systems. This hormone has been synthesized into various pharmaceutical forms—including the micronized plant-derived progesterone and synthetic versions called progestins—which act similarly to the natural form of progesterone. While the FDA hasn't approved progesterone therapy for PMS, many clinicians consider it useful for some women with severe symptoms. And the pharmaceutical forms of progesterone have received FDA-approval for the treatment of secondary amenorrhea (the disappearance of a woman's period after she's been menstruating regularly) and endometriosis (the presence of uterine tissue outside the uterus).

A progesterone deficiency has not been proven as a causal mechanism for PMS, and results of research using progesterone as a treatment for PMS haven't always been consistent. Some clinical studies have found dramatic PMS relief with the use of progesterone; others haven't. There is evidence that progesterone by-products vary in individual women, and it may also be that women react quite differently to progesterone preparations. One by-product might stimulate fluid retention in a particular woman, while another may relieve anxiety and tension. In fact, large doses of progesterone have been shown to have a calming effect in both men and women.

Proponents of progesterone treatment claim that because of the oral form's identical chemical structure to the form that naturally resides in a woman's body, the drug is generally well tolerated, produces few side effects, and provides therapeutic benefits. There are few side effects from micronized progesterone, beyond mild sedation or drowsiness, and it has not been linked with fetal abnormalities if it's used during pregnancy. What isn't known, however, is what effect continued use of progesterone treatment has on breast, vaginal, or cervical tissues. Current contraindications include liver dysfunction, known or suspected cancer, genital bleeding of unknown cause, and blood-clotting disorders. Because peanut oil is often used as the carrier agent in transdermal creams, women who are allergic to peanuts should not use these.

Progesterone therapy comes in many different forms, including oral capsules, a transdermal cream, vaginal or rectal suppositories, or a sublingual liquid (which is dropped under the tongue for immediate absorption). Micronized progesterone—which is simply progesterone that is broken up into very small particles—is the oral form of the natural progesterone that's produced by women's bodies. Most of the transdermal creams that are available without a prescription are advertised to include wild yam, a plant with progesterone-like properties. But in order for the active ingredient to bind with progesterone receptors, its structure must be altered in a laboratory process that's similar to what any pharmaceutical compound would go through. Some wild yam creams do contain micronized progesterone USP, which is therapeutic grade progesterone, so these may be of some benefit (keep in mind: OTC progesterone creams should contain about 450 mg. of progesterone per ounce; below this amount, they are not effective). Wild yam creams that don't contain progesterone are likely to be useless because they're not biologically available—in other words, your body cannot transform extract of wild yam into progesterone.

Natural progesterone can be readily absorbed when administered sublingually, intranasally, subdermally, intramuscularly, vaginally, and by rectal suppository. Oral administration of progesterone, once considered to be biologically inactive due to its rapid deterioration, has been modified through micronization or dissolution in oils that make it more readily absorbable. Micronized progesterone is available in the following forms and is prescribed for one to two weeks before menstruation:

- **Oral capsules:** The powdered form must be encapsulated by a local pharmacist or a mail-order pharmacy and requires a prescription from a licensed health-care provider. These can be taken one to three times per day, depending on the dosage in the capsule.

- **Transdermal creams or lotions:** These are available over-the-counter in health-food stores and pharmacies. The creams and lotions can be applied to the skin once or twice per day.

- **Suppositories:** These can be administered rectally or vaginally for rapid absorption. The suppositories must be compounded by a local pharmacist or obtained from a mail-order pharmacy with a prescription.

- **Sublingual liquids:** Available through mail-order sources and pharmacies, these usually require a prescription. The liquid is dropped under the tongue for immediate absorption (since it bypasses the digestive tract where it would be broken down by enzymes). These need to be taken frequently, up to six times per day.

- **Gels:** A 4 percent and an 8 percent micronized progesterone gel with a mineral-oil base are commercially available. These have received FDA approval for use as progesterone supplementation for assisted reproductive technology and for secondary amenorrhea. The gel is applied into the vagina.

- **Injections:** Intramuscular injections—in which progesterone is injected directly into a muscle—are available but these aren't recommended due to their invasive nature.

During the perimenopausal transition, women are likely to experience extreme ups and downs of hormones. Unlike the menopausal and postmenopausal periods when both estrogen and progesterone are low, estrogen is high during the perimenopause and progesterone is either absent (if a woman isn't ovulating) or low (if she's ovulating inadequately or has higher amounts of estrogen). This is when women are likely to experience their first hot flashes, night sweats, and sleep problems, especially during the premenstrual and menstrual phases of their cycles. These symptoms typically increase in frequency as the ovaries continue to sputter, releasing wildly fluctuating amounts of estrogen and progesterone.

One way to balance the relatively high levels of estrogen that occur during this time is to use natural, micronized progesterone or synthetic progestin, as recommended by Jerilynn Prior, M.D., an endocrinologist at the University of British Columbia in Vancouver, Canada. This mode of therapy is often used when a woman has a heavy menstrual flow, periods that come too close together, or an increase in cells that line the uterus (which is called endometrial hyperplasia). For these conditions, Dr. Prior recommends a six-month course of treatment with oral micronized progesterone in a dose of 300 mg. at bedtime or medroxyprogesterone (Provera) in a dose of 10 mg. per day for 16 days of the menstrual cycle. Of course, you will need a prescription from your health-care provider, who should supervise you during the treatment.

Oral Contraceptives:

A number of researchers have found that temporarily suppressing ovulation can reduce both PMS and postpartum depression in women who have been properly diagnosed with either condition. Birth-control pills may be an especially appealing option for women who typically experience symptoms that begin at ovulation, who experience marked premenstrual pain—pelvic pain, cramps, or menstrual migraines, for example—or who are having perimenopausal symptoms along with PMS, especially if they need to choose a contraceptive method anyway. Any low-dose oral contraceptive, containing estrogen and progestin, will suppress ovarian function, thereby preventing ovulation. The standard regimen is for three weeks of hormones and one week off hormones to allow for menstruation. If pelvic pain or cyclical headaches are part of the package of PMS symptoms, continuous administration of the pill is necessary.

For most women, a regimen of low-dose oral contraceptives, containing estrogen and progestin, is safe, even for women over age 35. Some of the more commonly recommended low-dose oral contraceptives include Alesse, Brevicon, Loestrin 1/20 or 1.5/30, Modicon, Norinyl 1+35 or 1+50, Ortho-Novum 1/35 and 1/50, Tri-Levlin, and Yasmin. (You should not consider using the Pill, however, if you are a smoker, have high blood pressure, cancer, or a history of liver disease.) Be forewarned, though, that while use of oral contraceptives can reduce PMS symptoms, they can also cause other symptoms. Some women who take the Pill experience fluid retention, weight gain, breakthrough bleeding (or midcycle spotting), or an intensification of migraine headaches or fibrocystic breast changes. In a study I conducted at the Oregon Health Sciences University in Portland, we also found that about 20 percent of women with PMS had their symptoms intensify while they were on the Pill. Although we did not determine the mechanism, these women appeared to have a sensitivity to synthetic ovarian hormones and reacted adversely to them. Unfortunately, there is no test to predict how you will respond to the hormones in oral contraceptives. The only way to find the right pill for you—or find out if there is one—is through trial and error.

Other Drugs That Block Ovulation:

When it comes to suppressing ovarian function, there are options besides oral contraceptives. Synthetic androgens—Danazol, Synarel, and Lupron, for example—block ovulation by interfering with the normal development of follicles (or eggs). In two PMS treatment studies, researchers administered these drugs via nasal spray or injection and found that women experienced marked relief of physical or pain symptoms and variable mood changes. The drawback to these, however, is that they have significantly more unpleasant side effects than oral contraceptives do—and they are much more expensive. Synthetic androgens can cause weight gain and unwanted hair growth, and while many women notice an increased libido or sexual arousal due to the effects of androgens on the brain, this typically goes hand-in-hand with an increase in aggressive feelings, similar to the premenstrual turmoil pattern of symptoms. But if you have another good reason for using these medications—if you're prone to endometriosis or ovarian cysts, for example—you also may find that the severity of your PMS diminishes.

Another drug called bromocriptine is often prescribed for women with breast pain. It's a dopamine receptor agonist that prohibits the production of prolactin, a hormone that stimulates breast development and milk production after pregnancy. The results of research, however, have been mixed: Some controlled studies have reported improvement in both mood and somatic symptoms when bromocriptine has been used for PMS while others have failed to support these findings. Side effects are common and include nausea, vomiting, and headaches.

There are no hard-and-fast rules for when to consider using a medication for PMS—nor are there any for which formulas are likely to be right for you. But if you continue to experience severe premenstrual symptoms even after your PMS plan is in full swing, you may want to consider using a medication as well. If your mood symptoms are continuing to send you on an emotional roller coaster, you may want to consider taking either micronized progesterone or one of the SSRI antidepressants. While the SSRI drugs appear to lessen both the depressive and anxiety symptoms, micronized progesterone acts more as an anti-anxiety agent, which means it may be better suited to the turmoil cluster of symptoms (tension, irritability, anger, feeling out of control, and the like). If you seem to be getting hit by the one-two punch of PMS and perimenopausal symptoms, this combination of symptoms also may be more responsive to micronized progesterone. If you aren't sensitive to synthetic hormones and you're in the market for contraception, the birth control pill may help decrease the mood, pain, and other physical symptoms that haven't been completely relieved by the PMS plan strategies.

Regardless of which medication you try, you may find that you can take a lower dose when you combine medication with the lifestyle changes from your PMS plan. In my research, we found that women who took SSRI antidepressants could take a lower dose if they combined it with their PMS plan. Other women found that they could discontinue taking antidepressants or anti-anxiety drugs after their PMS plans were well established. We also found that some women experienced fewer side effects with birth control pills when they were taking the regular daily multivitamin and mineral supplements and the PMS formula supplements.

The only way to find out which combination of protocols will do the trick is to experiment with different strategies until you find the magic medley that works for you. (Of course, if you are trying to get pregnant, you will want to be cautious about using any drug treatment; with the exception of micronized progesterone, none of these medications should be used during pregnancy.) Usually, you will need to try any of these medications for at least two or three menstrual cycles to be able to gauge the effects on your symptoms and to give your body a chance to overcome any side effects. At that point, if you need to adjust the dosage, you may need a couple of additional months to be able to judge the effects fairly.

13

Complicating Conditions

Though her PMS began in her teen years, the menstrual cycle wasn't always a source of distress for Grace, 39, a marketing manager. Some years were better than others. But once she reached her late thirties, the severe headaches, body aches, insomnia, irritability, depression, and trouble concentrating would often last for eight days. Her symptoms had become debilitating. The emotional and cognitive changes were the hardest to bear, especially during the winter months when her sense of well-being took a nosedive. "PMS drained me of energy and initiative and it interfered with my ability to function on many levels," she notes. "My negative mental state sometimes overwhelmed me. Mostly, I didn't like myself very much when I was premenstrual."

In an effort to gain control over her incapacitating symptoms, Grace made various changes to her diet. After two months, she stopped taking the PMS formula vitamins because they gave her digestive distress but continued taking a daily multivitamin and mineral supplement and added a B-complex vitamin. She also began walking and doing yoga regularly, used progressive muscle relaxation and various calming strategies, relied on thought-changing exercises to talk herself out of bad moods, and made an effort to improve her communication style, particularly with her husband and colleagues.

While these measures made a considerable difference in relieving her headaches, body discomfort, irritability, and concentration problems, Grace continued to experience depressive feelings, fatigue, and insomnia for the better part of the month. Her doctor suspected she was struggling with depression and perhaps also seasonal affective disorder (SAD)—mood changes that occur with the seasons—and prescribed Prozac. Her mood and sleep problems lifted and within a few months, she reduced her dosage. About that time, she also realized that marital problems had been compounding her symptoms so she and her husband began going to marriage counseling. Three months into it, Grace stopped taking Prozac altogether because her sense of well-being had increased substantially. All she was left with were two to three days of mild premenstrual blues, which she could handle.

Unfortunately, there's no law of nature that says that women can suffer from only one health condition at a time. The reality is, premenstrual symptoms or full-blown PMS may coexist with other conditions such as depression, anxiety disorders, asthma, migraines, and thyroid disorders, in what health professionals often refer to as dual diagnoses. Many of these conditions can actually increase in severity during the menstrual cycle, particularly in the premenstrual phase. Michelle Harrison, M.D., a leading expert on PMS, has labeled this process Premenstrual Magnification (PMM, for short). When a woman has both PMS and PMM, it's as if the two conditions are superimposed on her menstrual cycle.

The primary difference between the two phenomena is this: With PMS, symptoms occur only during the premenstrual phase and disappear within a day or two of menstrual bleeding; with PMM, symptoms are likely to be present to some degree all month long but they worsen during the premenstrual phase and gradually improve once a woman's period starts. But if she hasn't been diagnosed with the underlying condition, it can be difficult to extricate PMM from the PMS picture. That's why we asked you to plot "The Best of Times, Worst of Times Graph" in Chapter Three—to see in graphic form exactly what's going on with your cyclical symptoms. Without charting their symptoms in this fashion, many women simply don't make the link between flare-ups of other health conditions and the hormonal fluctuations that are associated with premenstrual changes. And if you haven't been diagnosed with the underlying problem, you may have thought your symptoms simply reflected PMS when they actually suggest there's a more complex mystery to be unraveled. If it turns out that some of the symptoms you thought were premenstrual actually exist in milder form throughout the month, you may have another health condition that warrants evaluation and treatment by a health-care professional.

There isn't a single explanation for why PMM occurs. The exact mechanism is different for each condition that becomes magnified premenstrually but the common denominator is likely to be the trickle-down effects of various hormonal fluctuations. What's more, there is some evidence of a slight downturn in immune function that occurs premenstrually. And, indeed, infections seem to occur more frequently or to worsen during the premenstrual phase of the menstrual cycle. Viral infections, such as herpes, seem to flare up at this time of the month, and some women report that they're more vulnerable to symptoms of colds or flu. Vaginal infections, especially yeast infections, often occur right before or during menstruation and have been found to be related to alterations in the normal vaginal pH level. The incidence of bladder infections increases during these phases for similar reasons.

In this chapter, we'll explore common conditions that can coexist with PMS—and help you figure out whether you might have one of these as well as premenstrual symptoms.

TROUBLE IN MIND

There is solid evidence that the menstrual cycle can exacerbate an underlying psychiatric disorder, trigger the expression of a psychiatric disorder, or synchronize the manifestation of such a disorder in a cyclical pattern. In fact, mood disorders—including major and mild depression, and bipolar disorders—can dwell quite harmoniously with PMS. So can anxiety disorders such as generalized anxiety disorder, panic attacks, phobias, obsessive-compulsive disorder, and post-traumatic stress disorder (PTSD).

About 25 percent of women will experience a mood disorder at some point in their lives, whereas 10 percent of men will. Yet, mood disorders in women are frequently undiagnosed and insufficiently treated due to the combination of somatic symptoms—such as pain, gastrointestinal distress, and fatigue—and depressive symptoms. It may be that clinicians often look for the wrong signs or miss atypical signs of a mood disorder. In a study of people in a primary care clinic, for example, 21 percent of those in the sample were subsequently diagnosed with a depressive disorder but only 1 percent described feelings of sadness or depression as the reason for their visit.

Similarly, many anxiety disorders go undiagnosed in women because physical symptoms predominate and laboratory tests are found to be normal. With panic disorder, for example, the original trigger may be far removed from the resulting anxiety or women may only describe symptoms such as dizziness, numbness, lightheadedness, or nausea. A woman with generalized anxiety disorder, by contrast, may describe exhaustion and sleep disturbances rather than her excessive worries or her inability to control her fears.

In a study, researchers from the Perinatal and Reproductive Psychiatry Clinical Research Program at Massachusetts General Hospital prospectively screened women who were not receiving treatment for a major psychiatric disorder (such as schizophrenia) for premenstrual dysphoric disorder (PMDD), or severe PMS. Depression was the most common mood disorder, affecting 13 percent of the women with PMDD, and panic disorder was found in 9 percent of the women with PMDD. This study also confirmed what other investigators have found—that mood disorders are twice as common as anxiety disorders and that for women, these disorders tend to become aggravated premenstrually.

What do these disorders have to do with the menstrual cycle? Plenty, it turns out. Depression and other mood disorders are believed to result from an imbalance in brain chemicals such as serotonin and norepinephrine. These neurotransmitters can be influenced by illnesses, prolonged physical or psychological stress, ovarian hormones, and genetic factors. Research has demonstrated that ovarian and stress hormones act on the brain and induce changes in all of the neurochemical pathways that are involved in mood and anxiety disorders. During the follicular phase, high levels of estrogen increase the amount of serotonin in the brain, acting as a natural antidepressant and mood stabilizer. Premenstrual surges of progesterone, on the other hand, reduce the effects of estrogen that were established in the follicular phase of the menstrual cycle and can produce feelings of distress and depression in some women. Complicating the picture, however, progesterone has been shown to have an anti-anxiety effect and appears to be related to decreased incidence of panic attacks in the mid-luteal phase when progesterone levels are high.

Women who have an underlying depressive disorder may be especially sensitive to these hormonal highs and lows. Moreover, in women with depression, the brain's ability to switch off the stress response seems to be impaired by the action of ovarian hormones on the brain. Under these conditions, it may take longer for a woman to return to a balanced state physically and emotionally.

Researchers at the Rockefeller University in New York City have described a process of allostatic loading, in which the brain becomes overwhelmed by stress and loses its physiologic ability to cope. The combination of stress and hormonal changes can serve as a double-whammy in this respect. When, month after month, a woman is faced with stressful life events as well as hormonal swings that affect her body and mind, the accumulation can become too much for the body and brain to bear. When certain events—whether it's a crisis at work, a sick child, or severe premenstrual misery—upset the precarious balance she has been maintaining, it's almost as if her brain registers "tilt." When this sort of chronic burden leads to overload, symptoms such as fatigue, headaches, anxiety, and depression can occur. It's as if her brain is sending out its own personal SOS.

Meanwhile, researchers at Columbia University in New York City have found that, in people with panic attacks, an abnormal firing of neurons and neurotransmitters occurs in an area of the brain that activates the stress response. These neurons fire randomly, seemingly without cause. People with panic disorders also appear to be especially sensitive to carbon dioxide changes in the blood, which can set off changes in the brain that are associated with the experience of emotion. So if women with PMS are breathing shallowly and upsetting the ratio of oxygen to carbon dioxide in their blood, this could trigger a panic attack or feelings of anxiety in those who are prone to them. Similarly, premenstrual hormonal fluctuations—by themselves—could trigger panic attacks in those who are susceptible.

ASTHMATIC PROBLEMS

Approximately 30 to 50 percent of women with asthma experience a premenstrual worsening of their asthma symptoms as well as a change in their breathing function, as measured by their peak expiratory flow rate (or PEFR). The underlying mechanism for this is poorly understood. One study in which women with premenstrual asthma were administered estrogen found improvement in asthma symptoms and pulmonary function, which suggests that the drop in estrogen that occurs during the premenstrual phase may play a role in this aggravation of symptoms. In several case study reports, however, oral contraceptives (which contain synthetic ovarian hormones) produced an exacerbation of asthma in premenopausal women with asthma.

Progesterone may play a role in the PMM of asthma, as well. Among the many sites of progesterone receptors are the nasal and pharyngeal passages and the lungs. When progesterone levels increase during the premenstrual phase, the receptors aren't able to bind as well with progesterone, which can make the lining of these respiratory passages more sensitive to irritants or changes in air quality. Depending upon a woman's personal vulnerability, this heightened sensitivity can lead to allergy flare-ups, asthma attacks, sinusitis, or sore throats.

But there seems to be a paradoxical response to the hormones that are produced by the ovaries compared to the hormones that are used in treatment. After all, progesterone treatment has also been found to reduce premenstrual provocation of asthma. Clearly, hormone levels seem to make a difference in premenstrual asthma flare-ups but whether the ups and downs of estrogen and progesterone help or aggravate the condition may depend on whether the source of those hormones is natural or synthetic as well as on a woman's personal sensitivity to these factors.

WHEN PMS GIVES YOU A HEADACHE

Nearly 20 million American women suffer from migraines—a recurring type of severe, throbbing headache—and about 60 percent of them experience a worsening of their migraines in association with their menstrual cycle. The term *menstrual migraine* is often used to describe hormonal headaches, even though these migraines can occur a few days before the onset of a woman's period. Estrogen withdrawal is thought to be a probable trigger for migraines in women who are susceptible. Susceptibility to menstrual migraines indicates that a woman is sensitive to hormonal changes; she also may be more sensitive to certain environmental stimuli. Moreover, recent research suggests that a complex impairment in the metabolism of prostaglandins and serotonin as well as changes in platelet function may play a significant role in menstrual migraine. But it isn't yet clear whether these changes occur on their own or as a result of changes in ovarian hormones such as estrogen and progesterone.

The mighty mineral magnesium may play a role in menstrual migraines, as well: Migraines, particularly in women, have been associated with deficits in magnesium levels in the brain and bloodstream. Recently, research by physiologists at the SUNY-Brooklyn Health Sciences Center has demonstrated that there are gender differences in the effects of reproductive hormones on magnesium levels in the brain. These scientists found that high levels of estrogen and progesterone—but not testosterone—significantly depleted ionized magnesium in blood vessels in the brain. This could result in spasms in these blood vessels along with reduced blood flow in the brain, both of which can trigger migraine headaches.

EPILEPSY

Approximately 1.1 million women of childbearing age in the U.S. have epilepsy. Many of these women experience changes in the frequency and severity of seizures that correspond to changes in their reproductive cycles—at puberty, during the menstrual cycle, with pregnancy, and at menopause. One-third to one-half of women with epilepsy have catamenial seizure patterns, which are characterized by an increase in seizures during particular phases of the menstrual cycle, usually the premenstrual phase and ovulation. In this case, estrogen, in particular, produces changes in a certain part of the brain that's related to cognitive function, which predisposes the synapses to the hyperexcitability that's associated with seizures. Indeed, in experimental models of epilepsy, estrogen has been found to have proconvulsant properties, whereas progesterone has anticonvulsant effects.

Since progesterone does exhibit anticonvulsant effects, seizures that occur during menstruation itself seem to be related to the decrease in progesterone that occurs just before the onset of a woman's period. Women with ovulatory cycles report a higher frequency of seizures during menstruation than during other phases of the menstrual cycle. Indeed, the most common precipitants that trigger or exacerbate seizures are stress, sleep deprivation, fatigue, and, for women, menstruation. Unfortunately, this reality may get worse before it gets better: Studies that have examined epilepsy in conjunction with menopause suggest that seizure activity decreases for some women after menopause but increases during the perimenopausal transition.

In addition, epilepsy can affect the reproductive system, inducing endocrine abnormalities, infertility, and sexual dysfunction, among other disorders. Unfortunately, the treatment for this condition can create similar problems. Anticonvulsant drugs may increase the risk of reproductive endocrine disorders in women with epilepsy, which could, in turn, cause more severe PMS.

WHEN PAIN STRIKES DEEP

Various forms of musculoskeletal pain—such as arthritis and fibromyalgia—can worsen during the premenstrual phase of a woman's cycle. Arthritis is a group of inflammatory disorders—which include osteoarthritis, a degenerative type, and rheumatoid arthritis, an autoimmune disorder—that lead to joint deterioration, stiffness, and pain. Fibromyalgia, by contrast, is a disorder of the tendons, muscles, and ligaments and does not involve the joints directly. While rheumatoid arthritis and fibromyalgia can occur in young women, osteoarthritis and other musculoskeletal conditions are more likely to be diagnosed at midlife.

Women may experience varying degrees of pain and soreness in the joints during the premenstrual phase but it usually disappears after their periods. The pain and discomfort that are associated with arthritis and fibromyalgia are likely to increase during the premenstrual period and during the perimenopause when hormone levels rise and fall with more extreme variability; in between, however, the discomfort doesn't disappear completely. Because many of the symptoms of fibromyalgia and rheumatoid arthritis overlap with the generalized pain, fatigue, and sleep disturbances that are associated with PMS, these conditions may go undiagnosed in women with moderate to severe PMS.

AN OUT-OF-WHACK THYROID

Thyroid problems are something of a silent epidemic: An estimated 13 million Americans, most of them women, suffer from an over- or underactive thyroid but 8 million of them don't even know it, according to the Thyroid Foundation of America. Indeed, many women of childbearing age may be wandering around for weeks, months, even years, feeling not quite their usual selves—and it may be because thyroid disorders are frequently overlooked in younger women. The thyroid is a small, butterfly-shaped gland in the lower part of the neck, one that affects nearly every organ in the body. Not only does the thyroid produce the major hormones that help regulate metabolism, but it also can affect your skin and hair, your muscle strength, your appetite, your mood and mental functioning, and your menstrual cycle.

Yet, because the symptoms of a thyroid problem are often quite subtle, a woman (or her doctor) might mistake the fatigue, forgetfulness, depressed mood, or weight gain that are associated with an underactive thyroid (called hypothyroidism) for the natural aging process. Or she may blame the sleep difficulties, nervousness, menstrual irregularities, increased appetite, or rapid heartbeat of an overactive thyroid (hyperthyroidism) on stress. (In my research, we found that almost one-third of women with PMM have an underlying thyroid problem, usually hypothyroidism.) In the early stages of either disorder, the symptoms may be mild—and could be confused with premenstrual symptoms. The difference is, they aren't likely to go away after the onset of menstrual bleeding. That's why blood tests, as well as a physical examination by a health-care provider, are used to diagnose thyroid disorders.

CYCLES OF DIGESTIVE DISTRESS

All menstruating women report that gastrointestinal symptoms such as abdominal pain and nausea are higher during their menstrual periods than at any other phase of the menstrual cycle. As it happens, a woman's stool consistency is also at its loosest during menstruation. While one-third of otherwise asymptomatic women may experience gastrointestinal symptoms at the time of menstruation, 50 percent of women with irritable bowel syndrome (IBS)—recurrent bouts of abdominal pain, diarrhea, and constipation—report a premenstrual increase in their symptoms. In a study comparing men and women who have IBS, researchers found that women more often reported nausea, alterations in taste and smell, greater food sensitivity, and muscle stiffness than men did; they also reported that these symptoms became more intense premenstrually. Similarly, women with functional bowel problems report more stomach pain, nausea, and diarrhea during their periods than women who don't have bowel problems.

Some investigators have found that gastrointestinal symptoms in women may be related to decreasing ovarian hormone levels or to other circulating agents—such as prostaglandins—that vary with the menstrual cycle. Of course, stress can also be an aggravating factor for digestive disorders. So if a woman experiences an increase in stress during the premenstrual phase of her cycle, that could trigger a bout of digestive distress, as well.

TIRED ALL THE TIME

Chronic fatigue is a debilitating condition that's accompanied by a constellation of symptoms that come and go, including muscle pain, a sore throat, tender lymph nodes, unusual headaches, and, of course, fatigue. These symptoms can resemble those of PMS but with chronic fatigue they don't necessarily ebb and flow in a predictable pattern. Clinical reports suggest that women with chronic fatigue do experience a premenstrual increase in pain and fatigue, which makes sense intuitively since changes in levels of estrogen and androgen hormones are associated with activation or suppression of the immune system. Levels of the stress hormone cortisol also increase in response to the decline in estrogen that occurs premenstrually, which can result in increased pain symptoms during the late premenstrual and menstrual phases or during the perimenopausal and postmenopausal periods when estrogen is declining.

While the cause of chronic fatigue is not well understood, the leading theory is that a virus, stress, or another trauma activates the immune system, which then remains in red-alert mode instead of slowing down as it would after an infection. As a result, a number of immune factors, some of which cause fatigue, remain in high concentrations. It is thought that chronic fatigue affects one out of every 1,000 adults.

A TRAUMATIC HISTORY

In some, severe instances, PMS may be a manifestation of post-traumatic stress disorder (PTSD), a specific form of anxiety that comes on after a traumatic event whose symptoms include intrusive thoughts, physiologic arousal, a sense of personal isolation, and disturbed sleep and concentration. In a recent study at UCSF, we found that an incredibly high percentage of women with severe PMS—twice as many women as in the general community—had a history of being sexually abused. It has been estimated that 12 to 40 percent of women in the U.S. have experienced childhood sexual abuse, whereas an estimated 13 to 27 percent of women have experienced sexual abuse as adults. Not surprisingly, 65 percent of the abused women in my study were found to have PTSD.

It's long been recognized that the physical and biochemical changes that occur with physical trauma have a wide-ranging impact on the body's tissues and set the stage for a chronic cycle of pain. Now, we are beginning to understand that emotional trauma can have similar effects. Increasingly sophisticated imaging techniques have allowed researchers to identify brain regions that are involved in the traumatic response. And several studies have shown structural and neurochemical changes in the parts of the brain that are associated with memory and emotions in women who've experienced childhood sexual assault.

Traumatic events evoke a stress response that, if continued long-term, can overwhelm a woman's self-regulatory capacity. As a result, she may experience PTSD. While research suggests that assault of all types carries the highest risk of subsequent PTSD, chronic emotional, physical, or sexual abuse or abuse that begins in childhood is the most severe form of stress, resulting in changes in brain biochemistry and PTSD. Recent research suggests that increased physiologic arousal—namely, a heightened stress response—and increased brain sensitivity to ovarian and adrenal hormones may limit the brain's ability to inhibit traumatic memories, which results in chronic anxiety and PTSD. As is the case with any form of severe stress, chronic anxiety and PTSD can, in turn, exacerbate PMS.

THE MIDLIFE TRANSITION

During the perimenopausal transition (approximately a four-year window between ages 40 and 58), ovulation begins to occur intermittently and menstrual cycles typically become irregular. With more extreme ups and downs of estrogen and sometimes progesterone, women are likely to experience daytime hot flashes, night sweats, fluid retention, pelvic or menstrual cramps, and an increased but often unpredictable menstrual flow. Do these symptoms point to PMS or perimenopause? The answer could be both. The truth is, these symptoms may or may not be related to the phase of your menstrual cycle; in either case, they are likely to be amplified by fluctuating levels of ovarian hormones, particularly estrogen, that occur in the perimenopause.

In studies at the University of Washington in Seattle, Nancy Woods, Ph.D., and colleagues found that women in the perimenopausal transition who also had PMS experienced similar symptom patterns to those of younger women with PMS. Like their younger counterparts, perimenopausal women with PMS have difficulty with anger management, concerns about self-control and social control, and higher life stress coupled with a heightened physiologic response to stress. Based on changes in blood pressure readings, women in the perimenopause who have PMS also do not appear to adapt as well to stress during the premenstrual phase as perimenopausal women who don't have PMS. Based on these findings, these researchers suggest that women with PMS may be at increased risk for hot flashes and night sweats, future depressive symptoms, and possibly cardiovascular changes as they experience the transition to menopause.

WHEN TO SUSPECT THAT MORE THAN PMS IS GOING ON

The patterns and severity of your symptoms are the best guide for sorting out whether you have PMM, severe PMS, or a dual diagnosis. Start with your primary health-care practitioner and bring along your PMS Tracking Charts as well as your menstrual and health history (from Chapter Three).

If you have been diagnosed with a health condition such as asthma, migraine headaches, or epilepsy, then you will want to consult your regular medical specialist or get a referral to a specialist from your primary-care doctor. What kind of specialist should you see? It depends, of course, on the condition. Many neurologists are trained to treat epilepsy or headaches, whereas pulmonologists have had extra training in asthma treatment. Gastroenterologists, on the other hand, have expertise in persistent digestive problems. And rheumatologists may be the ones to turn to if you continue to experience chronic fatigue or joint pain. For mood-related symptoms that continue after your menstrual period—especially if you have a history of depression or another mood or anxiety disorder—start with your primary-care provider or consult a mental health professional (a clinical psychologist, psychiatrist, licensed psychotherapist, psychiatric social worker or nurse practitioner, or a licensed marriage and family therapist).

Although there are no specific tests for either PMS or PMM, there are some laboratory tests that can be helpful in ruling out underlying problems. Simple blood tests can identify conditions such as anemia, thyroid disorders, diabetes, or hypoglycemia. And if you suspect that you are in the midst of the perimenopausal transition—which typically occurs in the early to late forties—then you may want to consult your primary-care practitioner for hormonal tests and a gynecological evaluation.

Of course, both premenstrual symptoms and the existing condition will require independent treatments. In some instances, with effective treatment of the underlying condition, the premenstrual symptoms will decrease in severity and not require their own treatment. On the other hand, by following your personalized PMS plan, you may be able to prevent or decrease premenstrual flare-ups of the underlying condition.

The bottom line: When a woman's premenstrual symptoms aren't adequately relieved by lifestyle modifications or other treatments that are designed for PMS, it's time to act like a detective and do some further investigating. It may be that you have another health condition that is worsening, thanks to hormonal fluctuations, or one that is exacerbating the actual symptoms of PMS. In such instances, the two conditions may need to be treated in tandem. That may be the only way a woman can truly regain her physical and emotional equilibrium and maintain it month after month.

Epilogue:

Taking Charge

ow that you've come to the end of the book, take a moment to congratulate yourself for trying to take charge of your symptoms—and, hence, your life. What you've been doing all this time, probably without even realizing it, is befriending your body, working with it—instead of against it—to achieve a state of greater well-being throughout the month. You've learned how to make connections between your symptoms and your behavior or lifestyle choices. You've experimented with different remedies that cater to your personal symptoms. And you've made a conscious effort to keep yourself on a more even emotional keel. What you've also done, in the process, is to elevate your health habits to a higher plane, which will undoubtedly enhance your health. After all, the self-care steps that are recommended in this book really create a roadmap to Wellville.

As Janice, 40, the arts consultant you first met in Chapter Seven, notes, "I feel so much lighter after making these changes. I'm not carrying around so much 'head garbage.' Instead of worrying about all the 'what if's,' I turn it around and think 'what's the worst thing that could happen?' Then, I'll take a deep breath, drink a glass of water, do the Lion yoga pose in front of the mirror and laugh at myself. I never thought I'd be laughing when I'm premenstrual."

Just because you've swung into action, though, that doesn't mean that your PMS plan is perfect. It's not supposed to be. Perfection implies an immutable state of excellence but the fact of the matter is, the menstrual cycle is anything but a fixed process. On the contrary, it's a dynamic process with many shifting characteristics so your personal PMS solution should evolve as your cycles and symptoms do. Besides, your menstrual cycle is not going to stop (until menopause, that is) so you will have plenty of chances to fine-tune or even reinvent your PMS plan through the months and years. Don't be afraid to tinker with it when the inclination strikes. This is your plan: Own it, shape it, make it work for you.

Of course, there may be times when you feel as though you're taking five giant steps forward in managing your premenstrual symptoms or your own daily world, only to take two or three steps back. Rest assured: This is quite normal. The dance of progress doesn't always take a predictable or linear course. Setbacks are likely to occur. Or, you might make rapid progress for a spell, only to find yourself stuck on a plateau for a few months. When these things happen, it's important to consider what you can learn from these experiences. Remind yourself that a lapse in progress doesn't have to lead to a collapse of your plan. Try to appreciate small changes. Let yourself feel proud of what you've accomplished so far. And try to anticipate your positive future. If you are patient and keep practicing the healthful measures you've embraced, you can and will make it farther along the path to PMS relief.

That's a lesson countless women learned from their experiences with the PMS Symptom Management Program at UCSF. As Naomi, 34, the occupational therapist you first met in Chapter Six, told me in the program's final days, "Of course, it's not all perfect but I give myself a lot more credit now. I have my fallback procedures for the difficult times and I talk to myself. I'll look at what I did right the previous week instead of focusing on what I didn't do and then I'll look at my calendar for the next two weeks and figure out a new schedule. I keep learning from what I'm doing, and that makes me feel good."

Like Naomi, the medical community has come a long way in understanding women's health from biological, psychological, and social perspectives. And researchers are continuing to investigate treatments that may be helpful for PMS. Premenstrual symptoms have come out of the closet—and so have relief measures. The strategies you've read about in this book place the care in your hands, which is where it belongs. Armed with reliable, up-to-date, accessible information and strategies, you are in a good position to take charge of managing your premenstrual symptoms and general well-being, even if that means seeking additional help—from your family, your friends, or from medical professionals—when necessary. By empowering yourself, you'll be more effective in the world around you. You're in your own good hands—trust them, along with the rest of your body and your mind, to guide you toward feeling better every day and every month.

Glossary

Aldosterone: A hormone that's secreted by the adrenal glands that helps control blood pressure and regulate the body's salt and water balance.

Autonomic nervous system: The part of the nervous system that controls bodily functions—such as beating of the heart, sweating, intestinal movements, and so on—that are involuntary or seemingly automatic. The autonomic nervous system actually consists of two parts—the sympathetic and the parasympathetic nervous systems. For the most part, the sympathetic system revs up activity in the body—increasing the heart and breathing rate in the face of stress or danger, for example. The parasympathetic system generally has the opposite effect; this is the system that predominates during sleep, for example. Most of the time, the two systems counterbalance each other.

Central nervous system: This is the overall term for the brain and the spinal cord. The general role of the central nervous system (CNS) is to receive sensory information from organs—including the eyes, ears, and receptors throughout the body—and to analyze this information and launch an appropriate motor response such as moving a muscle.

Corpus luteum: The tissue in the ovary that forms at the site of a ruptured egg after ovulation; it secretes the hormone progesterone to prepare the womb for implantation of a fertilized egg. If implantation doesn't occur, the corpus luteum degenerates. If implantation does occur, the corpus luteum continues to produce progesterone until the fourth month of pregnancy, at which time the placenta takes over this function.

Cortisol: A steroid hormone produced by the adrenal glands, cortisol is vital to the normal stress response (a.k.a., the fight-or-flight response). It is also essential for proper carbohydrate metabolism in the body.

DHEA (dehydroepiandrosterone): A hormone that's secreted by the adrenal glands, often as part of the stress response. Technically, DHEA is an androgen (a male hormone) that can be converted to estradiol (one of the three main estrogens) and testosterone.

Dopamine: This neurotransmitter—one of many chemical messengers that allow nerve cells to "talk" to each other—plays an important role in parts of the brain that control movement and mood.

Dysmenorrhea: This means painful menstruation, characterized by menstrual cramps, nausea, vomiting, faintness, and other forms of discomfort that occur before or during a woman's period. The exact cause of this menstrual discomfort isn't known but a leading theory is that it's due to excessive production of—or high sensitivity to—prostaglandins, hormonelike substances that stimulate contractions of the uterus and other smooth muscles.

Endorphins: Often called the body's natural painkillers, endorphins are a group of substances that are produced in the brain and have a similar chemical structure to morphine; hence, they relieve pain. They are also believed to control the body's response to stress, affect mood and feelings of well-being, and influence the release of various hormones. Exercise, particularly the vigorous variety, has been found to raise levels of endorphins.

Estrogen: An umbrella term for a group of hormones that are produced by the ovaries and adrenal glands and are essential for normal female sexual development as well as functioning of the reproductive system.

Fight-or-flight response: The physiological response that occurs when the sympathetic branch of the autonomic nervous system is aroused—namely, when you are dealing with a real or perceived danger, threat, or other source of stress. The adrenal glands release the stress hormones epinephrine (a.k.a., adrenaline) and norepinephrine which lead to increased heart rate, breathing, blood pressure, and blood flow to the muscles to make the body better able to fight or flee the threat. This physiological stress response can also be ignited by constant stress and anxiety.

Follicle-stimulating hormone (FSH): A hormone that's produced by the pituitary gland in the brain to stimulate follicles (or eggs) inside the ovary to develop and secrete more estrogen.

Follicular phase: The first half of a woman's menstrual cycle, beginning with the first day of her period and ending with ovulation. During this time, the hormones estrogen and progesterone cause changes in the lining of the uterus and the follicle-stimulating hormone (FSH) stimulates the growth of several eggs in the ovaries.

Homeostasis: A dynamic physiological process in which the body's internal systems maintain their own state of balance or environmental equilibrium, even as external conditions fluctuate. This mechanism applies to blood pressure, body temperature, blood sugar levels, and the body's acid-base balance, among other factors.

Luteal phase: The second half of the menstrual cycle, the luteal phase occurs after ovulation and lasts until the start of a woman's next period. During this time, the corpus luteum is formed and the uterus is prepared for the possibility of pregnancy. Premenstrual symptoms can occur any time during the luteal phase but are more likely during the latter days.

Luteinizing hormone (LH): A hormone that's released by the pituitary gland and triggers ovulation, the formation of the corpus luteum, and the synthesis of other hormones in the body.

Menarche: This is the technical term for the onset of menstruation, usually around the age of 12 or 13 or within a few years after the first physical signs of puberty appear.

Menopause: The permanent cessation of menstruation, usually between the ages of 45 and 55, which occurs as a result of a declining production of estrogen by the ovaries. Symptoms such as hot flashes, night sweats, vaginal dryness, and decreased sex drive are the most common experiences that may occur during menopause; the good news is, premenstrual symptoms generally disappear after menopause.

Menstrual cycle: The monthly sequence of events in a nonpregnant woman of reproductive age in which an egg is released by the ovary every four weeks or so until menopause. If the egg is not fertilized, the cycle continues and the uterus sheds its lining at menstruation. If the egg is fertilized and becomes implanted in the womb, pregnancy begins.

Menstruation: The shedding of the lining of the uterus, which results in menstrual bleeding every month, as long as a woman doesn't become pregnant.

Neurotransmitters: Chemical messengers that relay impulses from one nerve cell to another (or to a muscle cell) in the brain and in the body. Important neurotransmitters include acetylcholine, dopamine, norepinephrine, and serotonin.

Norepinephrine: A stress hormone that's secreted by the adrenal glands, norepinephrine helps constrict blood vessels (thereby leading to increased blood pressure), slow down heart rate, and increase the depth and rate of breathing. The hormone is also released as a neurotransmitter by certain nerve endings in the sympathetic nervous system.

Ovary: One member of a pair of almond-shaped glands that are located on either side of the uterus, just below the opening of the fallopian tube. Each ovary contains numerous follicles within which egg (or ovum) cells develop. The ovaries also produce the female sex hormones estrogen and progesterone as well as small amounts of androgen hormones (such as testosterone).

Ovulation: The monthly development and release of an egg (or ovum) from a follicle within the ovary.

Perimenopause: A period of approximately four or five years before menopause when a woman's menstrual cycles become irregular, thanks to erratic ovulation patterns and widely fluctuating hormone levels that result from aging ovaries. Many body functions—including sleep, memory, mood, energy, immune action, skin health, and sexual function—are affected by these fluctuations.

Premenstrual dysphoric disorder (PMDD): A severe form of PMS that's characterized as a major mood disorder in the latest *Diagnostic and Statistical Manual* (DSM-IV), the bible of psychiatric diagnoses. The symptoms are largely the same as those in premenstrual syndrome (PMS) but with PMDD they are so severe that they interfere with a woman's ability to function.

Premenstrual magnification (PMM): A cyclical flare-up of an underlying condition, one that worsens during the premenstrual phase. Unlike the usual pattern of PMS, however, these symptoms may ease in severity at other times of the month but may not go away completely.

Premenstrual phase: The period of time lasting from seven to 14 days before the onset of a woman's period, the premenstrual phase occurs during the luteal phase—or second half—of a woman's menstrual cycle.

Premenstrual syndrome (PMS): A diagnostic term that's used to describe cyclical recurrences of distressing physical, emotional, and behavioral symptoms that often affect a woman's personal health and sense of well-being. Symptoms—from breast tenderness or water retention to mood swings or irritability—typically occur during the week or two before menstruation and continue until the onset of a woman's period; they generally disappear within the first two days of menstruation.

Progesterone: A female sex hormone that is produced in the ovaries during the second half of the menstrual cycle, progesterone causes the lining of the uterus to thicken to prepare for pregnancy (specifically, the implantation of a fertilized egg).

Prolactin: A hormone secreted by the pituitary gland that stimulates milk production after childbirth as well as production of progesterone by the ovaries.

Prostaglandins: Hormone-like substances that are produced in various body tissues including the uterus, brain, and kidneys, prostaglandins can stimulate contractions of smooth muscle such as the uterus, causing menstrual-related pain and discomfort. The primary weapons against prostaglandins are nonsteroidal anti-inflammatory drugs (NSAIDs), which block the production of prostaglandins in the body.

Seasonal affective disorder (SAD): A type of depression that is associated with the change of seasons and fluctuations in the intensity of natural light and the duration of daylight hours during the year. Bright-light therapy has been found to help those who suffer from SAD.

Serotonin: Though it is a compound that is present in many tissues of the body, serotonin is most famous as a neurotransmitter in the brain, one that is involved in the regulation of mood and sleep, among other factors. Low levels of serotonin have been associated with depression.

Sympathetic nervous system: See autonomic nervous system.

Tryptophan: An essential amino acid that is a building block for the neurotransmitter serotonin. Foods that are rich in tryptophan include canned tuna or canned salmon, meat, low-fat cottage cheese, skim milk, and lima beans.

Tyrosine: An amino acid that is a precursor for the neurotransmitters dopamine, epinephrine, and norepinephrine, tyrosine can help improve concentration and mood. Good dietary sources of tyrosine include cheddar cheese, almonds, sesame seeds, roasted turkey, plain low-fat yogurt, and peas.

Uterus: The hollow, muscular organ in a woman's pelvic cavity in which a fertilized egg becomes implanted and in which the developing fetus is nourished during pregnancy. (It is also called the womb.) The uterus is lined with a special tissue, called endometrium, which undergoes changes during the menstrual cycle; if pregnancy doesn't occur, the endometrium is shed during menstruation, resulting in menstrual bleeding.

APPENDIX 1

References and Further Reading

Appendix 1:

References and Further Reading

These references include the best articles, books, and research to support content in chapters 1–13 or for further reading.

Chapter One: The Puzzle of PMS

Anson, O. "Exploring the Biopsychosocial Approach to Premenstrual Experiences." *Social Science and Medicine* 49 (1999): 67–80.

Asso, Doreen. *The Real Menstrual Cycle.* New York: Wiley & Sons, 1983.

Asso, D., and Magos, A. "Psychological and Physiological Changes in Severe Premenstrual Syndrome." *Biological Psychology* 33 (1992): 115–32.

Bloch, M., Schmidt, P. J., Su, T. P., Tobin, M. B., and Rubinow, D. R. "Pituitary-adrenal Hormones and Testosterone Across the Menstrual Cycle in Women with Premenstrual Syndrome and Controls." *Biological Psychiatry* 43 (1998): 897–903.

The Boston Women's Health Book Collective. *The New Our Bodies Ourselves: A Book By and For Women.* New York: Touchstone/Simon & Schuster, 1992.

Busch, C., Costa, P., et al. "Severe Perimenstrual Symptoms: Prevalence and Effects on Absenteeism and Health Care Seeking in a Non-clinical Sample." *Women and Health* 14 (1988): 59–74.

Deuster, P. A., Adera, T., and South-Paul, J. "Biological, Social, and Behavioral Factors Associated with Premenstrual Syndrome." *Archives of Family Medicine* 8 (1999): 122–8.

Endicott, J. "The Epidemiology of Perimenstrual Psychological Symptoms." *Acta Psychiatrica Scandinavica* 104 (2001): 110–6.

Figert, A. E. *Women and the Ownership of PMS: The Structuring of a Psychiatric Disorder.* New York: Aldine De Gruyter, 1986.

Freeman, E. W. "Premenstrual Syndrome: Current Perspectives on Treatment and Etiology." *Current Opinions in Obstetrics and Gynecology* 9 (1997):147–53.

Gurevich, M. "Rethinking the Label: Who Benefits from the PMS Construct?" *Women and Health* 23 (1995): 67–98.

Halbreich, U. "Premenstrual Syndromes: Closing the 20th Century Chapters." *Current Opinions in Obstetrics and Gynecology* 11 (1999): 265–70.

Halbreich, U. "Menstrually Related Disorders—Towards Interdisciplinary International Diagnostic Criteria." *Cephalalgia* 17 (1997): 1–4.

Lewis, L. L., Greenblatt, E. M., Rittenhouse, C. A., Veldhuis, J. D., and Jaffe, R. B. "Pulsatile Release Patterns of Luteinizing Hormone and Progesterone in Relation to Symptom Onset in Women with Premenstrual Syndrome." *Fertility and Sterility* 64 (1995): 288–92.

Mortola, J. F. "Premenstrual Syndrome—Pathophysiologic Considerations." *New England Journal of Medicine* 338 (1998): 256–7.

Parlee, M. B. "Media Treatment of Premenstrual Syndrome." In *Premenstrual Syndrome: Ethical and Legal Implications in a Biomedical Perspective,* edited by B. E. Ginsburg and B. F. Carter, pp. 189–205. New York: Plenum, 1987.

Rapkin, A. J., Morgan, M., Goldman, L., Brann, D. W., Simone, D., and Mahesh, V. B. "Progesterone Metabolite Allopregnanolone in Women with Premenstrual Syndrome." *Obstetrics and Gynecology* 90 (1997): 709–14.

Redei, E., and Freeman, E. W. "Daily Plasma Estradiol and Progesterone Levels Over the Menstrual Cycle and Their Relation to Premenstrual Symptoms." *Psychoneuroendocrinology* 20 (1995): 259–67.

Rubinow, D. R., Schmidt, P. J., and Roca, C. A. "Estrogen-Serotonin Interactions: Implications for Affective Regulation." *Biological Psychiatry* 44 (1998): 839–50.

Rubinow, D. R., Schmidt, P. J., and Roca, C. A. "Hormone Measures in Reproductive Endocrine-Related Mood Disorders: Diagnostic Issues." *Psychopharmacology Bulletin* 34 (1998): 289–90.

Rubinow, D. R, and Schmidt, P. J. "The Neuroendocrinology of Menstrual Cycle Mood Disorders." *Annals of the New York Academy of Science* 771 (1995): 648–59.

Rubinow, D. R, and Schmidt, P. J. "The Treatment of Premenstrual Syndrome—Forward Into the Past." *New England Journal of Medicine* 332 (1995): 1574–5.

Schmidt, P. J., Nieman, L. K., Danaceau, M. A., Adams, L. F., and Rubinow, D. R. "Differential Behavioral Effects of Gonadal Steroids in Women with and in Those without Premenstrual Syndrome." *New England Journal of Medicine* 338 (1998): 209–16.

Seippel, L., and Backstrom, T. "Luteal-phase Estradiol Relates to Symptom Severity in Patients with Premenstrual Syndrome." *Journal of Clinical Endocrinology and Metabolism* 83 (1998): 1988–92.

Severino, S., and Moline, M. *Premenstrual Syndrome.* New York: Guilford, 1989.

Sommer, B. "Stress and Menstrual Distress." *Journal of Human Stress* 4 (1978): 5–47.

Sundstrom, I., Backstrom, T., Wang, M., Olsson, T., Seippel, L., and Bixo, M. "Premenstrual Syndrome, Neuroactive Steroids and the Brain." *Gynecological Endocrinology* 13 (1999): 206–20.

Sundstrom, I., Andersson, A., Nyberg, S., Ashbrook, D., Purdy, R. H., and Backstrom, T. "Patients with Premenstrual Syndrome Have a Different Sensitivity to a Neuroactive Steroid During the Menstrual Cycle Compared to Control Subjects." *Neuroendocrinology* 67 (1998): 126–38.

Taylor, D., Woods, N., et al. "An Explanatory Model of Perimenstrual Negative Affect." In *Menstruation, Health and Illness*, edited by D. Taylor and N. Woods, pp. 103–118. New York: Hemisphere, 1991.

Treolar, A. E., Boynton, R. E., Borghild, G. B., and Brown, B. W. "Variation of the Human Menstrual Cycle Through Reproductive Life." *International Journal of Fertility* 12 (1991): 77–126.

Van Goozen, S. H., Frijda, N. H., Wiegant, V. M., Endert, E., and Van de Poll, N. E. "The Premenstrual Phase and Reactions to Aversive Events: A Study of Hormonal Influences on Emotionality." *Psychoneuroendocrinology* 21 (1996): 479–97.

Voda, A. M. "The Tremin Trust: An Intergenerational Research Program on Events Associated with Women's Menstrual and Reproductive Lives." In *Menstruation, Health and Illness*, edited by D. Taylor and N. F. Woods, pp. 5–18. Washington, DC: Hemisphere/Taylor & Francis, 1991.

Voda, A. M., and Mansfield, P. K. "Menstrual Bleeding Patterns in Premenopausal Women." In *Mind-Body Rhythmicity: A Menstrual Cycle Perspective*, edited by N. Woods. Seattle: Hamilton & Cross, 1994.

Woods, N. F. "Premenstrual Symptoms: Another Look." *Public Health Reports* Jul–Aug; Suppl (1987): 106–12.

Woods, N. F., Most, A., and Dery, G. K. "Prevalence of Perimenstrual Symptoms." *American Journal of Public Health* 72 (1982): 1257–64.

Zita, J. N. "The Premenstrual Syndrome: 'Dis-easing' the Female Cycle." *Hypatia* 3 (1988): 77–79.

Chapter Two: The Ages and Stages of PMS

Bancroft, J. "The Menstrual Cycle and the Well Being of Women." *Social Science and Medicine* 41 (1995): 785–91.

Buckley, Thomas, and Gottlieb, Alma, eds. *Blood Magic: The Anthropology of Menstruation*. Berkeley: University of California Press, 1988.

Chrisler, J. C., Johnson, I., Champagne, N., and Preston, K. "Menstrual Joy: The Construct and Its Consequences." *Psychology of Women Quarterly* 18 (1994): 375–387.

Chuong, C. J., and Burgos, D. M. "Medical History in Women with Premenstrual Syndrome." *Journal of Psychosomatic Obstetrics and Gynaecology* 16 (1995): 21–7.

Cleckner-Smith, C. S., Doughty, A. S., and Grossman, J. A. "Premenstrual Symptoms. Prevalence and Severity in an Adolescent Sample." *Journal of Adolescent Health* 22 (1998): 403–8.

Dalton, K. "The Influence of Menstruation on Health and Disease." *Proceedings of the Royal Society of Medicine* 57 (1964): 262–264.

Dalton, K. *Once a Month: The Premenstrual Syndrome*. Pomona, CA : Hunter House, 1979.

Dan, A., and Lewis, L., eds. *Menstrual Health in Women's Lives*. Chicago: University of Illinois Press, 1992.

Delaney, J., Lupton, M., et al. "The Storm Before the Calm: The Premenstrual Syndrome." In *The Curse: The Cultural History of Menstruation*, edited by J. Delaney, M. Lupton, and E. Toth, 92–104. New York: E. P. Dutton, 1976.

Dennerstein, L., Gotts, G., Brown, J. B., Morse, C. A., Farley, T. M., and Pinol, A. "The Relationship Between the Menstrual Cycle and Female Sexual Interest in Women with PMS Complaints and Volunteers." *Psychoneuroendocrinology* 19 (1994): 293–304.

Frank, R. "The Hormonal Causes of Premenstrual Tension." *Archives of Neurologic Psychiatry* 26 (1931): 1031–1033.

Freeman, E. W., Schweizer, E., and Rickels, K. "Personality Factors in Women with Premenstrual Syndrome." *Psychosomatic Medicine* 57 (1995): 453–9.

Freeman, E. W., Rickels, K., Schweizer, E., and Ting, T. "Relationships Between Age and Symptom Severity Among Women Seeking Medical Treatment for Premenstrual Symptoms." *Psychological Medicine* 25 (1995): 309–15.

Futterman, L. A., Jones, J. E., et al. "Severity of Premenstrual Symptoms in Relation to Medical/Psychiatric Problems and Life Experiences." *Perceptual and Motor Skills* 74 (1992): 787–799.

Glick, H., Endicott, J., and Nee, J. "Premenstrual Changes: Are They Familial?" *Acta Psychiatrica Scandanavica* 88 (1993): 149–55.

Janiger, O., Riffenburgh, M., and Kersh, M. "A Cross-Cultural Study of Premenstrual Symptoms." *Psychosomatics* 13 (1972): 226–235.

Markens, S. "The Problematic of Experience: A Political and Cultural Critique of PMS." *Gender and Society* 10 (1996): 42–58.

Martin, E. *The Woman in the Body: A Cultural Analysis of Reproduction.* Boston: Beacon, 1987.

Marvan, M. L., and Escobedo, C. "Premenstrual Symptomology: Role of Prior Knowledge About Premenstrual Syndrome." *Psychosomatic Medicine* 61 (1999): 163–7.

McMaster, J., Cormie, K., and Pitts, M. "Menstrual and Premenstrual Experiences of Women in a Developing Country." *Health Care for Women International* 18 (1997): 533–41.

Menke, E. "Menstrual Beliefs and Experiences of Mother-Daughter Dyads." In *Menarche*, edited by S. Golub, pp. 133–37. New York: Lexington, 1983.

Metcalf, M. G., and Livesey, J. H. "Distribution of Positive Moods in Women with the Premenstrual Syndrome and in Normal Women." *Journal of Psychosomatic Research* 39 (1995): 609–18.

Morse, C. A., Dudley, E., Guthrie, J., and Dennerstein, L. "Relationships Between Premenstrual Complaints and Perimenopausal Experiences." *Journal of Psychosomatic Obstetrics and Gynaecology* 19 (1998): 182–91.

Santoro, N., Rosenberg-Brown, J., Adel, T., and Skurnick, J. H. "Characterization of Reproductive Hormonal Dynamics in the Perimenopause." *Journal of Clinical Endocrinology and Metabolism* 81 (1996): 1495–1501.

Severy, L., Thapa, S., Askew, I. L., and Glor, J. "Menstrual Experiences and Beliefs: A Multicountry Study of Relationships with Fertility and Fertility-Regulating Methods." *Women and Health* 20 (1993): 1–20.

Shuttle, P., and Redgrove, P. *The Wise Wound: Myths, Realities, and Meanings of Menstruation.* New York: Grove, 1986.

Stoltzman, S. M. "Menstrual Attitudes, Beliefs and Symptom Experiences of Adolescent Females, Their Peers, and Their Mothers." In *Culture, Society and Menstruation*, edited by V. L. Olesen, and N. F. Woods, pp. 97–114. Washington, DC: Hemisphere/Taylor & Francis, 1986.

Sugawara, M., Toda, M. A., Shima, S., Mukai, T., Sakakura, K., and Kitamura, T. "Premenstrual Mood Changes and Maternal Mental Health in Pregnancy and the Postpartum Period." *Journal of Clinical Psychology* 53 (1997): 225–32.

Taylor, D., and Woods, N. F., eds. *Menstruation, Health & Illness.* New York: Taylor & Francis, 1991.

Walker, A. *The Menstrual Cycle: This pernicious mischief.* London: Routledge, 1997.

Woods, N. F. "Socialization and Social Context: Influence on Perimenstrual Symptoms, Disability, and Menstrual Attitudes." *Health Care for Women International* 7 (1986): 115–29.

Woods, N. F., Dery, G. K., and Most, A. "Recollections of Menarche, Current Menstrual Attitudes, and Perimenstrual Symptoms." *Psychosomatic Medicine* 44 (1982): 285–93.

World Health Organization. "A Cross-Cultural Study of Menstruation: Implications for Contraceptive Development and Use." *Studies in Family Planning* 12 (1981): 3–16.

Chapter Three: Getting in Touch with Your Symptoms

Futterman, L., Jones, J., et al. "Assessing Premenstrual Syndrome Using the Premenstrual Experience Assessment." *Psychological Reports* 63 (1988): 19–34.

Mitchell, E., Woods, N., Lentz, M., and Taylor, D. "Recognizing PMS When You See It: Criteria for PMS Sample Selection." In *Menstruation, Health and Illness*, edited by D. Taylor and N. F. Woods, pp. 89–118. Washington, DC: Taylor & Francis, 1991.

Mitchell, E., Lentz, M., et al. "Methodologic Issues in the Definition of Perimenstrual Symptoms." In *Menstrual Health in Women's Lives*, edited by A. Dan and L. Lewis. Urbana, IL: University of Illinois Press, 1992.

Mitchell, E. S., Woods, N. F., and Lentz, M. J. "Differentiation of Women with Three Perimenstrual Symptom Patterns." *Nursing Research* 43 (1994): 25–30.

Moos, R. (1969). "Typology of Menstrual Cycle Symptoms." *American Journal of Obstetrics & Gynecology*, 103: 390–402.

Rubinow, D. R., and Roy-Byrne, P. "Premenstrual Syndromes: Overview from a Methodologic Perspective." *American Journal of Psychiatry* 41 (1984): 163–72.

Shaver, J. F., and Woods, N. F. "Concordance of Perimenstrual Symptoms Across Two Cycles." *Research in Nursing and Health* 8 (1985): 313–9.

Taylor, D. "Evaluating Therapeutic Change in Symptom Severity at the Level of the Individual Woman Experiencing Severe PMS." *Image: Journal of Nursing Scholarship* 26 (1994): 25–33.

Woods, N. F., Mitchell, E. S., and Lentz, M. "Premenstrual Symptoms: Delineating Symptom Clusters." *Journal of Women's Health and Gender-Based Medicine* 8 (1999): 1053–62.

Chapter Four: The PMS Diet

Abraham, G., and Hargrove, J. "Effect of Vitamin B6 on Premenstrual Symptomology in Women with Premenstrual Tension Syndrome: A Double-Blind Crossover Study." *Infertility* 3 (1980): 155.

Barnard, N. D., Scialli, A. R., Hurlock, D., and Bertron, P. "Diet and Sex-Hormone Binding Globulin, Dysmenorrhea, and Premenstrual Symptoms." *Obstetrics and Gynecology* 95 (2000): 245–50.

Bendich, A. "The Potential for Dietary Supplements to Reduce Premenstrual Syndrome (PMS) Symptoms." *Journal of American College of Nutrition* 19 (2000): 3–12.

Chakmakjian, Z. H., Higgins, C. E., and Abraham, G. E. "The Effect of a Nutritional Supplement, Optivite for Women, on Premenstrual Tension Syndromes." *Journal of Applied Nutrition* 37 (1985): 12–7.

Christensen, L. "The Effect of Carbohydrates on Affect." *Nutrition* 13 (1997): 503–14.

Chuong, C. J., Dawson, E. B., and Smith, E. R. "Vitamin E Levels in Premenstrual Syndrome." *American Journal of Obstetrics and Gynecology* 163 (1990): 1591–5.

De Souza, M. C., Walker, A. F., Robinson, P. A., and Bolland, K. "A Synergistic Effect of a Daily Supplement for 1 Month of 200 Mg Magnesium Plus 50 Mg Vitamin B6 for the Relief of Anxiety-Related Premenstrual Symptoms: A Randomized, Double-Blind, Crossover Study." *Journal of Women's Health and Gender-Based Medicine* 9 (2000): 131–9.

Facchinetti, F., Borella, P., Sances, G., Fioroni, L., Nappi, R. E., and Genazzani, A. R. "Oral Magnesium Successfully Relieves Premenstrual Mood Changes." *Obstetrics and Gynecology* 78 (1991): 177–81.

Heaney, R. P., Dowell, S. D., Bierman, J., Hale, C. A., and Bendich, A. "Absorbability and Cost Effectiveness in Calcium Supplementation." *Journal of the American College of Nutrition* 20 (2001): 239–46.

Kleijnen, J., Ter-Riet, G., and Knipschild, P. "Vitamin B6 in the Treatment of the Premenstrual Syndrome—A Review." *British Journal of Obstetrics and Gynaecology* 97 (1990): 847–52.

Macdougall, M. "Poor-Quality Studies Suggest That Vitamin B6 Use Is Beneficial in Premenstrual Syndrome." *Western Journal of Medicine* 172 (2000): 245.

Michener, W., Rozin, P., Freeman, E., and Gale, L. "The Role of Low Progesterone and Tension as Triggers of Perimenstrual Chocolate and Sweets Craving: Some Negative Experimental Evidence." *Physiology and Behavior* 67 (1999): 417–20.

Mira, M., Stewart, P. M., and Abraham, S. F. "Vitamin and Trace Element Status in Premenstrual Syndrome." *American Journal of Clinical Nutrition* 47 (1988): 636–41.

Muneyvirci-Delale, O., Nacharaju, V. L., Altura, B. M., and Altura, B. T. "Sex Steroid Hormones Modulate Serum Ionized Magnesium and Calcium

Levels Throughout the Menstrual Cycle in Women." *Fertility and Sterility* 69 (1998): 958–62.

Posaci, C., Erten, O., Uren, A., and Acar, B. "Plasma Copper, Zinc and Magnesium Levels in Patients with Premenstrual Tension Syndrome." *Acta Obstetrica et Gynecologica Scandanavica* 73 (1994): 452–5.

Reeves, B. D., Garvin, J. E., and McElin, T. W. "Premenstrual Tension: Symptoms and Weight Changes Related to Potassium Therapy." *American Journal of Obstetrics and Gynecology* 109 (1971): 1036–41.

Rosenstein, D. L., Ryschon, T. W., Niemela, J. E., Elin, R. J., Balaban, R. S., and Rubinow, D. R. "Skeletal Muscle Intracellular Ionized Magnesium Measured by 31P-NMR Spectroscopy Across the Menstrual Cycle." *Journal of the American College of Nutrition* 14 (1995): 486–90.

Rosenstein, D. L., Elin, R. J., Hosseini, J. M., Grover, G., and Rubinow, D. R. "Magnesium Measures Across the Menstrual Cycle in Premenstrual Syndrome." *Biological Psychiatry* 35 (1994): 557–61.

Rossignol, A., and Bonnlander, H. "Caffeine-Containing Beverages, Total Fluid Consumption, and Premenstrual Syndrome." *American Journal of Public Health* 80 (1990): 1106–10.

Sayegh, R., Schiff, I., Wurtman, J., Spiers, P., McDermott, J., and Wurtman, R. "The Effect of a Carbohydrate-Rich Beverage on Mood, Appetite, and Cognitive Function in Women with Premenstrual Syndrome." *Obstetrics and Gynecology* 86 (1995): 520–8.

Stewart, A. "Clinical and Biochemical Effects of Nutritional Supplementation on the Premenstrual Syndrome." *Journal of Reproductive Medicine* 32 (1987): 435–4.

Thys-Jacobs, S. "Micronutrients and the Premenstrual Syndrome: The Case for Calcium." *Journal of the American College of Nutrition* 19 (2000): 220–7.

Thys-Jacobs, S., Ceccarelli, S., Bierman, A., Weisman, H., Cohen, M. A., and Alvir, J. "Calcium Supplementation in Premenstrual Syndrome: A Randomized Crossover Trial." *Journal of General Internal Medicine* 4 (1989): 183–9.

Walker, A. F., De Souza, M. C., Vickers, M. F., Abeyasekera, S., Collins, M. L., and Trinca, L. A. "Magnesium Supplementation Alleviates Premenstrual Symptoms of Fluid Retention." *Journal of Women's Health* 7 (1998): 1157–65.

Wallin, M. S., and Rissanen, A. M. "Food and Mood: Relationship Between Food, Serotonin, and Affective Disorders." *Acta Psychiatrica Scandanavica* 377 (1994): 36–40.

Ward, M. W., and Holimon, T. D. "Calcium Treatment For Premenstrual Syndrome." *Annals of Pharmacotherapy* 33 (1999): 1356–8.

Wurtman, R. J., and Wurtman J. J. "Brain Serotonin, Carbohydrate-Craving, Obesity and Depression." *Obesity Research* 3 (1995): 477S–480S.

Wyatt, K. M., Dimmock, P. W., Jones, P. W., and Shaughn O'Brien, P. M. "Efficacy of Vitamin B-6 in the Treatment of Premenstrual Syndrome: Systematic Review." *British Medical Journal* 318 (1999): 1375–81.

Chapter Five: Exercising Your Options

Aganoff, J. A., and Boyle, G. J. "Aerobic Exercise, Mood States and Menstrual Cycle Symptoms." *Journal of Psychosomatic Research* 38 (1994): 183–92.

Bibi, K. W. "The Effects of Aerobic Exercise on Premenstrual Syndrome Symptoms." *Dissertation Abstracts International* 56 (1995): 6678.

Carmack, C. L., Boudreaux, E., Amaral-Melendez, M., Brantley, P. J., and de Moor, C. "Aerobic Fitness and Leisure Physical Activity as Moderators of the Stress-Illness Relation." *Annals of Behavioral Medicine* 21 (1999): 251–7

Choi, P. Y., and Salmon, P. "Symptom Changes Across the Menstrual Cycle in Competitive Sportswomen, Exercisers and Sedentary Women." *British Journal of Clinical Psychology* 34 (1995): 447–60.

Choi, P. Y., and Salmon, P. "Stress Responsivity in Exercisers and Non-Exercisers During Different Phases of the Menstrual Cycle." *Social Science and Medicine* 41 (1995): 769–77.

DiLorenzo, T. M., Bargman, E. P., Stucky-Ropp, R., Brassington, G. S., Frensch, P. A., and LaFontaine, T. "Long-term Effects of Aerobic Exercise on Psychological Outcomes." *Preventative Medicine* 28 (1999): 75–85.

Dishman, R. K. "Brain Monoamines, Exercise, and Behavioral Stress: Animal Models." *Medicine and Science in Sports and Exercise* 29 (1997): 63–74.

Dishman, R. K., Renner, K. J., White-Welkley, J. E., Burke, K. A., and Bunnell, B. N. "Treadmill Exercise Training Augments Brain Norepinephrine Response to Familiar and Novel Stress." *Brain Research Bulletin* 52 (2000): 337–42.

Fox, K. R. "The Influence of Physical Activity on Mental Well-Being." *Public Health and Nutrition* 2 (1999): 411–8.

Giacomoni, M., Bernard, T., Gavarry, O., Altare, S., and Falgairette, G. "Influence of the Menstrual Cycle Phase and Menstrual Symptoms on Maximal Anaerobic Performance." *Medicine and Science in Sports and Exercise* 32 (2000): 486–92.

Hightower, M. "Effects of Exercise Participation on Menstrual Pain and Symptoms." *Women and Health* 26 (1997): 15–27.

Lemos, D. "The Effects of Aerobic Training on Women Who Suffer From Premenstrual Syndrome." *Dissertation Abstracts International* 52 (1991): 563.

Prior, J. C., Vigna, Y., Sciarretta, D., Alojada, N., and Schulzer, M. "Conditioning Exercise Decreases Premenstrual Symptoms: A Prospective Controlled 6-Month Trial." *Fertility and Sterility* 47 (1987): 402–8.

Scully, D., Kremer, J., Meade, M. M., Graham, R., and Dudgeon K. "Physical Exercise and Psychological Well Being: A Critical Review." *British Journal of Sports Medicine* 32 (1998): 111–20.

Steege, J. F., and Blumenthal, J. A. "The Effects of Aerobic Exercise on Premenstrual Symptoms in Middle Aged Women: A Preliminary Study." *Journal of Psychosomatic Research* 37 (1993): 127–33.

Chapter Six: The Role of Relaxation

Anisman, H., and Zacharko, R. "Depression as a Consequence of Inadequate Neurochemical Adaptation in Response to Stressors." *British Journal of Psychiatry* 160 (1992): 36–43.

Brown, M., and Harrington, S. "A Comparative Analysis of Stress in Women With Varying Levels of Premenstrual Symptomatology." *Communicating Nursing Research* 19 (1986): 10–14.

Cahill, C. A. "Differences in Cortisol, a Stress Hormone, in Women With Turmoil-Type Premenstrual Symptoms." *Nursing Research* 47 (1998): 278–84.

Goodale, I. L., Domar, A. D., and Benson, H. "Alleviation of Premenstrual Syndrome Symptoms with the Relaxation Response." *Obstetrics and Gynecology* 75 (1990): 649–55.

Leserman, J., Li, Z., Hu, Y. J., and Drossman, D. A. "How Multiple Types of Stressors Impact on Health." *Psychosomatic Medicine* 60 (1998): 175–181.

Maddocks, S. E., and Reid, R. L. "The Role of Negative Life Stress and PMS: Some Preliminary Findings." In *Menstrual Health in Women's Lives*, edited by A. J. Dan and L. L. Lewis, pp. 38–51. Chicago: University of Illinois Press, 1992.

Reichlin, S., Abplanalp, J. M., Labrum, A. H., Schwartz, N., Sommer, B., and Taymor, M. "The Role of Stress in Female Reproductive Dysfunction." *Journal of Human Stress* 5 (1979): 38–45.

Sapolsky, R. M. "Why Stress Is Bad For Your Brain." *Science* 273 (1996): 749–750.

Woods, N. F., Lentz, M. J., Mitchell, E. S., Heitkemper, M., Shaver, J., and Henker, R. "Perceived Stress, Physiologic Stress Arousal, and Premenstrual Symptoms: Group Differences and Intra-Individual Patterns." *Research in Nursing and Health* 21 (1998): 511–23.

Woods, N. F., Lentz, M. J., Mitchell, E. S., and Heitkemper, M. "Luteal Phase Ovarian Steroids, Stress Arousal, Premenses Perceived Stress, and Premenstrual Symptoms." *Research in Nursing and Health* 21 (1998): 129–42.

Woods, N. F., Lentz, M. J., Mitchell, E. S., and Kogan, H. "Arousal and Stress Response Across the Menstrual Cycle in Women with Three Perimenstrual Symptom Patterns." *Research in Nursing and Health* 17 (1994): 99–110.

Woods, N. F., Most, A., and Longenecker, G. D. "Major Life Events, Daily Stressors, and Perimenstrual Symptoms." *Nursing Research* 34 (1985): 263–7.

Woods, N. F. "Relationship of Socialization and Stress to Perimenstrual Symptoms, Disability, and Menstrual Attitudes." *Nursing Research* 34 (1985): 145–9.

Woods, N. F., Dery, G. K., and Most, A. "Stressful Life Events and Perimenstrual Symptoms." *Journal of Human Stress* 8 (1982): 23–31.

Chapter Seven: Giving Your Mindset a Makeover

Berman, K. F., Schmidt, P. J., Rubinow, D. R., Danaceau, M. A., Van Horn, J. D., Esposito, G., Ostrem, J. L., and Weinberger, D. R. "Modulation of Cognition-Specific Cortical Activity by Gonadal Steroids: A Positron-Emission Tomography Study in Women." *Proceedings of the National Academy of Sciences USA* 94 (1997): 8836–41.

Blake, F., Salkovskis, P., Gath, D., Day, A., and Garrod, A. "Cognitive Therapy for Premenstrual Syndrome: A Controlled Trial." *Journal of Psychosomatic Research* 45 (1998): 307–18.

Christensen, A. P., and Oei, T. P. "The Efficacy of Cognitive Behaviour Therapy in Treating Premenstrual Dysphoric Changes." *Journal of Affective Disorders* 33 (1995): 57–63.

Drossman, D. A., Leserman, J., Li, Z., Keefe, F., Hu, Y. J., and Toomey, T. C. "Effects of Coping on Health Outcome Among Women with Gastrointestinal Disorders." *Psychosomatic Medicine* 62 (2000): 309–17.

Fink, G., Sumner, B. E., Rosie, R., Grace, O., and Quinn, J. P. "Estrogen Control of Central Neurotransmission: Effect on Mood, Mental State, and Memory." *Cellular and Molecular Neurobiology* 16 (1996): 325–44.

Fontaine, K. R., and Seal, A. "Optimism, Social Support, and Premenstrual Dysphoria." *Journal of Clinical Psychology* 53 (1997): 243–7.

Fontana, A. M., and Badawy, S. "Perceptual and Coping Processes Across the Menstrual Cycle: An Investigation in a Premenstrual Syndrome Clinic and a Community Sample." *Behavioral Medicine* 22 (1997): 152–9.

Hamilton, J., Alagna, S., and Sharpe, A. "Cognitive Approaches to Understanding and Treating Premenstrual Depression." In *Premenstrual Syndrome*, edited by H. Ofofsky, pp. 69–84. Washington, DC: American Psychiatric Press, 1985.

Keenan. P. A., Lindamer, L. A., and Jong, S. K. "Menstrual Phase-Independent Retrieval Deficit in Women with PMS." *Biological Psychiatry* 38 (1995):369–77.

Kirkby, R. J. "Changes in Premenstrual Symptoms and Irrational Thinking Following Cognitive-Behavioral Coping Skills Training." *Journal of Consulting and Clinical Psychology* 62 (1994): 1026–32.

Man, M. S., MacMillan, I., Scott, J., and Young, A. H. "Mood, Neuropsychological Function and Cognitions in Premenstrual Dysphoric Disorder." *Psychological Medicine* 29 (1999): 727–33.

McEwen, B. S. "Protective and Damaging Effects of Stress Mediators." *Seminars in Medicine of Beth Israel Deaconess Medical Center* 338 (1998):171–9.

Meichenbaum, D. "Changing Conceptions of Cognitive Behavior Modification: Retrospect and Prospect." *Journal of Consulting and Clinical Psychology* 61 (1993): 202–4.

Meichenbaum, D., and Novaco, R. "Stress Inoculation: A Preventative Approach." *Issues in Mental Health Nursing* 7 (1985): 419–35.

Morgan, M., Rapkin, A. J., D'Elia, L., Reading, A., and Goldman, L. "Cognitive Functioning in Premenstrual Syndrome." *Obstetrics and Gynecology* 88 (1996): 961–6.

Morse, G. "Positively Reframing Perceptions of the Menstrual Cycle Among Women with Premenstrual Syndrome." *Journal of Obstetric, Gynecologic, and Neonatal Nursing* 28 (1999): 165–74.

Schacter, D. L. "The Seven Sins of Memory. Insights from Psychology and Cognitive Neuroscience." *American Psychologist* 54 (1999): 182–203.

Wolkowitz, O. M., Weingartner, H., Rubinow, D. R., Jimerson, D., Kling, M., Berretini, W., Thompson, K., Breier, A., Doran, A., and Reus, V. I. "Steroid Modulation of Human Memory: Biochemical Correlates." *Biological Psychiatry* 33 (1993): 744–6.

Chapter Eight: Managing Your Time

Emmett, R: *The Procrastinators Handbook*. New York: Walker & Co., 2000.

Lee, K., Lentz, M., Taylor, D., Mitchell, E., and Woods, N. F. "Fatigue as a Response to Environmental Demands in Women's Lives." *Image: Journal of Nursing Scholarship* 26 (1994): 149–54.

Levine, R. V., Lynch, K., Miyake, K., and Lucia, M. "The Type A City: Coronary Heart Disease and the Pace of Life." *Journal of Behavioral Medicine* 12 (1989): 509–12.

Levine, R. V. "The Pace of Life." *Psychology Today* 20 (1989): 42–46.

Morgenstern, J. *Time Management from the Inside Out*. New York: Henry Holt, 2000.

Chapter Nine: The Relationship Dance of PMS
Brown, M., and Zimmer, P. "Personal and Family Impact of Premenstrual Symptoms." *Journal of Obstetric, Gynecological, Neonatal Nursing* 15 (1986): 31–38.

Clayton, A. H., Clavet, G. J., McGarvey, E. L., Warnock, J. K., and Weiss, K. "Assessment of Sexual Functioning During the Menstrual Cycle." *Journal of Sex and Marital Therapy* 25 (1999): 281–91.

Cortese, J., and Brown, M. A. "Coping Responses of Men Whose Partners Experience Premenstrual Symptomatology." *Journal of Obstetric, Gynecologic, and Neonatal Nursing* 18 (1989): 405–12.

Ekholm, U., and Backstrom, T. "Influence of PMS on Family, Social Life, and Work Performance." *International Journal of Health Services* 24 (1994): 629–647.

Fradkin, B., and Firestone, P. "Premenstrual Tension, Expectancy, and Mother-Child Relations." *Journal of Behavioral Medicine* 9 (1986): 245–59.

Lee, K., and Rittenhouse, C. A. "Health and Perimenstrual Symptoms: Health Outcomes for Employed Women Who Experience Perimenstrual Symptoms." *Women and Health* 19 (1992): 65–77.

Mansfield, P. K., Hood, K. E., and Henderson, J. "Women and Their Husbands: Mood and Arousal Fluctuations Across the Menstrual Cycle and Days of the Week." *Psychosomatic Medicine* 51 (1989): 66–80.

Mills, S. "The Impact of Stress on PMS Severity for Women in Couple Relationships." In *Mind-Body Rhythmicity: A Menstrual Cycle Perspective*, edited by N. Woods. Seattle: Hamilton & Cross, 1994.

Orth-Gomier, K., Wamala, S. P. Horsten, M., Schenck-Gustafson, K., Schneiderman, N., and Mittleman, M.A. "Marital Stress Worsens Prognosis in Women with Coronary Disease: The Stockholm Coronary Risk Study." *JAMA* 284 (2000): 3008–14.

Tannen, D. *That's Not What I Meant!* New York: Ballantine, 2000.

Tannen, D. *You Just Don't Understand: Women and Men in Conversation.* New York: Ballantine, 1990.

Taylor, D., and Bledsoe, L. "PMS, Stress and Social Support: A Pilot Study and Therapeutic Hypotheses." In *Culture, Society, and Menstruation*, edited by V. Oleson and N. Woods. Washington, D.C.: Hemisphere, 1985.

Chapter Ten: Putting the Pieces Together
Morse, G. G. "Effect of Positive Reframing and Social Support on Perception of Perimenstrual Changes Among Women with PMS." *Health Care for Women International* 18 (1997): 175–93.

Taylor, D. "More Than Personal Change: Effective Elements of Symptom Management." *Nurse Practitioner Forum* 11 (2000): 1–10.

Taylor, D. "Effectiveness of Professional–Peer Group Treatment: Symptom Management for Women with PMS." *Research in Nursing and Health* 22 (1999): 496–511.

Chapter Eleven: Emerging Therapies for PMS

Berger, D., Schaffner, W., Schrader, E., Meier, B., and Brattstrom, A. "Efficacy of Vitex Agnus Castus L. Extract Ze 440 in Patients with Pre-Menstrual Syndrome (PMS)." *Archives of Gynecology and Obstetrics* 264 (2000): 150–3.

Callender, K., McGregor, M., Kirk, P., and Thomas, C. S. "A Double-Blind Trial of Evening Primrose Oil in the Premenstrual Syndrome: Nervous Symptom Subgroup." *Human Psychopharmacology* 3 (1988): 57–61.

Chapman, E. H., Angelica, J., Spitalny, G., and Strauss, M. "Results of a Study of the Homeopathic Treatment of PMS." *Journal of the American Institute of Homeopathy* 87 (1994): 14–21.

Collins, A., Cerin, A., Coleman, G., and Landgren, B. M. "Essential Fatty Acids in the Treatment of Premenstrual Syndrome." *Obstetrics and Gynecology* 81 (1993): 93–8.

Hardy, M. L. "Herbs of Special Interest to Women." *Journal of the American Pharmacological Association (Washington)* 40 (2000): 234–42.

Hernandez-Reif, M., Martinez, A., Field, T., Quintero, O., Hart, S., and Burman, I. "Premenstrual Symptoms Are Relieved by Massage Therapy." *Journal of Psychosomatic Obstetrics and Gynaecology* 21 (2000): 9–15.

Kleijnen, J. "Evening Primrose Oil." *British Medical Journal* 309 (1994): 824–5.

Lam, R. W., Carter, D., Misri, S., Kuan, A. J., Yatham, L. N., and Zis, A. P. "A Controlled Study of Light Therapy in Women with Late Luteal Phase Dysphoric Disorder." *Psychiatry Research* 86 (1999): 185–92.

Loch, E. G., Selle, H., and Boblitz, N. "Treatment of Premenstrual Syndrome with a Phytopharmaceutical Formulation Containing Vitex Agnus Castus." *Journal of Women's Health and Gender-Based Medicine* 9 (2000): 315–20.

London, R. S., Bradley, L., and Chiamori, N. Y. "Effect of a Nutritional Supplement on Premenstrual Symptomatology in Women with Premenstrual Syndrome: A Double-Blind Longitudinal Study." *Journal of the American College of Nutrition* 10 (1991): 494–9.

London, R. S., Sundaram, G. S., Murphy, L., and Goldstein, P. J. "The Effect of Alpha-Tocopherol on Premenstrual Symptomology: A Double-Blind Study." *Journal of the American College of Nutrition* 2 (1983): 115–22.

O'Hara, M. A., Kiefer, D., and Farrell, K. "A Review of 12 Commonly Used Medicinal Herbs." *Archives of Family Medicine* 7 (1998): 523–36.

Oleson, T., and Flocco, W. "Randomised Controlled Study of Premenstrual Symptoms Treated with Ear, Hand, and Foot Reflexology." *Acta Obstetrica et Gynecologica Scandanavica* 50 (1971): 331–7.

Parry, B. L., Berga, S. L., Mostofi, N., Klauber, M. R., and Resnick, A. "Plasma Melatonin Circadian Rhythms During the Menstrual Cycle and After Light Therapy in Premenstrual Dysphoric Disorder and Normal Control Subjects." *Journal of Biological Rhythms* 12 (1997): 47–64.

Parry, B. L, Hauger, R., Lin, E., Le Veau, B., Mostofi, N., Clopton, P. L., and Gillin, J. C. "Neuroendocrine Effects of Light Therapy in Late Luteal Phase Dysphoric Disorder." *Biological Psychiatry* 36 (1994): 356–64.

Pearlstein, T., and Steiner, M. "Non-Antidepressant Treatment of Premenstrual Syndrome." *Journal of Clinical Psychiatry* 61 (2000): 22–7.

Schellenberg, R. "Treatment for the Premenstrual Syndrome with Agnus Castus Fruit Extract: Prospective, Randomised, Placebo Controlled Study." *British Medical Journal* 322 (2001): 134–7.

Steinberg, S., Annable, L., Young, S. N., and Liyanage, N. "A Placebo-Controlled Clinical Trial of L-Tryptophan in Premenstrual Dysphoria." *Biological Psychiatry* 45 (1999): 313–20.

Stevinson, C., and Ernst, E. "Complementary/Alternative Therapies for Premenstrual Syndrome: A Systematic Review of Randomized Controlled Trials." *American Journal of Obstetrics and Gynecology* 185 (2001): 227–35.

Stevinson, C., and Ernst, E. "A Pilot Study of Hypericum Perforatum for the Treatment of Premenstrual Syndrome." *British Journal of Obstetrics and Gynecology* 107 (2000): 870–6.

Tamborini, A., and Taurelle, R. "Value of Standardized Ginkgo Biloba Extract (Egb 761) in the Management of Congestive Symptoms of Premenstrual Syndrome [French]." *Review of French Gynécology and Obstétrics* 88 (1993): 447–57.

Turner, S., and Mills, S. "A Double-Blind Clinical Trial on a Herbal Remedy for Premenstrual Syndrome: A Case Study." *Complementary and Therapeutic Medicine* 1 (1993): 73–7.

Van Zak, D. B. "Biofeedback Treatments for Premenstrual and Premenstrual Affective Syndromes." *International Journal of Psychosomatics* 41 (1994): 53–60.

Walsh, M. J., and Polus, B. I. "A Randomized, Placebo-Controlled Clinical Trial on the Efficacy of Chiropractic Therapy on Premenstrual Syndrome." *Journal of Manipulative and Physiological Therapies* 22 (1999): 582–5.

Yakir, M., Kreitler, S., Brzezinski, A., Vithoulkas, G., Oberbaum, M., and Bentwich, Z. "Effects of Homeopathic Treatment in Women with Premenstrual Syndrome: A Pilot Study." *The British Homeopathic Journal* 90 (2001): 148–53.

Chapter Twelve: Medicating Measures

Dimmock, P. W., Wyatt, K. M., Jones, P. W., and O'Brien, P. M. "Efficacy of Selective Serotonin-Reuptake Inhibitors in Premenstrual Syndrome: A Systematic Review." *Lancet* 356 (2000): 1131–6.

Freeman, E. W., Kroll, R., Rapkin, A., Pearlstein, T., Brown, C., Parsey, K., Zhang, P., Patel. H., and Foegh, M. "Evaluation of a Unique Oral Contraceptive In the Treatment of Premenstrual Dysphoric Disorder." *Journal of Women's Health and Gender-Based Medicine* 10 (2001): 561–9.

Freeman, E. W., Rickels, K., Sondheimer, S. J., and Polansky, M. "Differential Response to Antidepressants in Women with Premenstrual Syndrome/Premenstrual Dysphoric Disorder: A Randomized Controlled Trial." *Archives of General Psychiatry* 56 (1999): 932–9.

Freeman, E. W., Rickels, K., Sondheimer, S. J., and Polansky, M. "A Double-Blind Trial of Oral Progesterone, Alprazolam, and Placebo in Treatment of Severe Premenstrual Syndrome." *JAMA* 274 (1995): 51–7.

Freeman, E. W., Weinstock, L., Rickels, K., Sondheimer, S. J., and Coutifaris, C. "A Placebo-Controlled Study of Effects of Oral Progesterone on Performance and Mood." *British Journal of Clinical Pharmacology* 33 (1992): 293–8.

Halbreich, U., Rojansky, N., and Palter, S. "Elimination of Ovulation and Menstrual Cyclicity (with Danazol) Improves Dysphoric Premenstrual Syndromes." *Fertility and Sterility* 56 (1991): 1066–9.

Hamilton, J. A., Alagna, S. W., and Pinkel, S. "Gender Differences in Antidepressant and Activating Drug Effects on Self-Perceptions." *Journal of Affective Disorders* 7 (1984): 235–43.

Hammarback, S., and Backstrom, T. "Induced Anovulation as Treatment of Premenstrual Tension Syndrome." *Acta Obstetrica et Gynecologica Scandinavica* 67 (1988): 159–166.

Hart, K. E., and Hill, A. L. "Generalized Use of Over-the-Counter Analgesics: Relationship to Premenstrual Symptoms." *Journal of Clinical Psychology* 53 (1997): 197–200.

Magill, P. J. "Investigation of the Efficacy of Progesterone Pessaries in the Relief of Symptoms of Premenstrual Syndrome. Progesterone Study Group." *British Journal of General Practice* 45 (1995): 589–93.

Martorano, J. T., Ahlgrimm, M., and Colbert, T. "Differentiating Between Natural Progesterone and Synthetic Progestins: Clinical Implications for

Premenstrual Syndrome and Perimenopause Management." *Comprehensive Therapy* 24 (1998): 336–9.

Moline, M. L. "Pharmacologic Strategies for Managing Premenstrual Syndrome." *Clinical Pharmacology* 12 (1993): 181–96.

Schmidt, P. J., Grover, G. N., and Rubinow DR. "Alprazolam in the Treatment of Premenstrual Syndrome. A Double-Blind, Placebo-Controlled Trial." *Archives of General Psychiatry* 50 (1993): 467–73.

Simon, J. A. "Micronized Progesterone: Vaginal and Oral Uses." *Clinical Obstetrics and Gynecology* 38 (1995): 902–14.

Steiner, M., Romano, S. J., Babcock, S., Dillon, J., Shuler, C., Berger, C., Carter, D., Reid, R., Stewart, D., Steinberg, S., and Judge, R. "The Efficacy of Fluoxetine in Improving Physical Symptoms Associated with Premenstrual Dysphoric Disorder." *British Journal of Obstetrics and Gynaecology* 108 (2001): 462–8.

Sundstrom, I., Nyberg, S., Bixo, M., Hammarback, S., and Backstrom, T. "Treatment of Premenstrual Syndrome with Gonadotropin-Releasing Hormone Agonist in a Low Dose Regimen." *Acta Obstetrica et Gynecologica Scandinavica* 10 (1999): 891–9.

Wang, M., Hammarback, S., Lindhe, B. A., and Backstrom, T. "Treatment of Premenstrual Syndrome by Spironolactone: A Double-Blind, Placebo-Controlled Study." *Acta Obstetrica et Gynecologica Scandinavica* 74 (1995): 803–8.

Wyatt, K., Dimmock, P., Jones, P., Obhrai, M., and O'Brien, S. "Efficacy of Progesterone and Progestogens in Management of Premenstrual Syndrome: Systematic Review." *British Medical Journal* 323 (2001): 776–80.

Yonkers, K. A., Halbreich, U., Freeman, E., Brown, C., Endicott, J., Frank, E., Parry, B., Pearlstein, T., Severino, S., Stout, A., Stone, A., and Harrison, W. "Symptomatic Improvement of Premenstrual Dysphoric Disorder with Sertraline Treatment. A Randomized Controlled Trial. Sertraline Premenstrual Dysphoric Collaborative Study Group." *JAMA* 24 (1997): 983–8.

Chapter Thirteen: Complicating Conditions

Ader, D. N., Shriver, C. D., and Browne, M. W. "Cyclical Mastalgia: Premenstrual Syndrome or Recurrent Pain Disorder?" *Journal of Psychosomatic Obstetrics and Gynaecology* 20 (1999): 198–202.

American Psychiatric Association. *Diagnostic and Statistical Manual of Mental Disorders*. Washington D.C.: American Psychiatric Association, 1994.

Betrus, P. A., Elmore, S. K., Woods, N. F., and Hamilton, P. A. "Women and Depression." *Health Care for Women International* 16 (1995): 243–52.

Bancroft, J., and Rennie, D. "Perimenstrual Depression: Its Relationship to Pain, Bleeding, and Previous History of Depression." *Psychosomatic Medicine* 57 (1995): 445–52.

Breaux, C., Hartlage, S., and Gehlert, S. "Relationships of Premenstrual Dysphoric Disorder to Major Depression and Anxiety Disorders: A Re-Examination." *Journal of Psychosomatic Obstetrics and Gynaecology* 21 (2000): 17–24.

Caplan, Paula. *They Say You're Crazy: How the World's Most Powerful Psychiatrists Decide Who's Normal.* New York: Perseus Press 1996.

Chaturvedi, S. K., Chandra, P. S., Gururaj, G., Pandian, R. D., and Beena, M. B. "Suicidal Ideas During Premenstrual Phase." *Journal of Affective Disorders* 34 (1995): 193–9.

Denicoff, K. D., Joffe, R. T., Lakshmanan, M. C., Robbins, J., and Rubinow, D. R. "Neuropsychiatric Manifestations of Altered Thyroid State." *American Journal of Psychiatry* 147 (1990): 94–9.

Endicott, J. "History, Evolution, and Diagnosis of Premenstrual Dysphoric Disorder." *Journal of Clinical Psychiatry* 61 (2000): 5–8.

Endicott, J., Amsterdam, J., Eriksson, E., Frank, E., Freeman, E., Hirschfeld, R., Ling, F., Parry, B., Pearlstein, T., Rosenbaum, J., Rubinow, D., Schmidt, P., Severino, S., Steiner, M., Stewart, D. E., and Thys-Jacobs, S. "Is Premenstrual Dysphoric Disorder a Distinct Clinical Entity?" *Journal of Women's Health and Gender-Based Medicine* 8 (1999): 663–79.

Endicott, J. "The Menstrual Cycle and Mood Disorders." *Journal of Affective Disorders* 29 (1993): 193–200.

Facchinetti, F., Tarabusi, M., and Nappi, G. "Premenstrual Syndrome and Anxiety Disorders: A Psychobiological Link." *Psychotherapy and Psychosomatics* 67 (1998): 57–60.

Fisher, D. A. "Desideratum Dermatologicum—Cause and Control of Premenstrual Acne Flare." *International Journal of Dermatology* 39 (2000): 334–6.

Gehlert, S., Chang, C. H., and Hartlage, S. "Symptom Patterns of Premenstrual Dysphoric Disorder as Defined in the Diagnostic and Statistical Manual of Mental Disorders-IV." *Journal of Women's Health* 8 (1999): 75–85.

Girdler, S. S., Pedersen, C. A., and Light, K. C. "Thyroid Axis Function During the Menstrual Cycle in Women with Premenstrual Syndrome." *Psychoneuroendocrinology* 20 (1995): 395–403

Golding, J., and Taylor D. "Sexual Assault History and Premenstrual Distress in Two General Population Samples." *Journal of Women's Health* 5 (1996): 143–152.

Golding, J. M., Taylor, D., Menard, L., and King, M. J. "Prevalence of Sexual Abuse History in a Sample of Women Seeking Treatment for Premenstrual Syndrome." *Journal of Psychosomatic Obstetrics and Gynaecology* 21 (2000): 69–80.

Halbreich, U. "Premenstrual Dysphoric Disorders: A Diversified Cluster of Vulnerability Traits to Depression." *Acta Obstetrica et Gynecologica Scandinavica* 95 (1997): 169–76.

Halbreich, U. "Menstrually Related Disorders: What We Do Know, What We Only Believe That We Know, and What We Know That We Do Not Know." *Critical Review of Neurobiology* 9 (1995): 163–75.

Hamilton, J. A., and Gallant, S. J. "Debate on Late Luteal Phase Dysphoric Disorder." *American Journal of Psychiatry* 147 (1990): 1106–7.

Kendler, K. S., Karkowski, L. M., Corey, L. A., and Neale, M. C. "Longitudinal Population-Based Twin Study of Retrospectively Reported Premenstrual Symptoms and Lifetime Major Depression." *American Journal of Psychiatry* 155 (1998): 1234–40.

Kljakovic, M., and Pullon, S. "Allergy and the Premenstrual Syndrome (PMS)." *Allergy* 52 (1997): 681–3.

Larsson, C., and Hallman J. "Is Severity of Premenstrual Symptoms Related to Illness in the Climacteric?" *Journal of Psychosomatic Obstetrics and Gynaecology* 18 (1997): 234–43.

Lemieux, A. M., and Coe, C. L. "Abuse-Related Posttraumatic Stress Disorder: Evidence for Chronic Neuroendocrine Activation in Women." *Psychosomatic Medicine* 57 (1995): 105–15.

North American Menopause Society. "Clinical Challenges of Perimenopause: Consensus Opinion of the North American Menopause Society." *Menopause* 7 (2000): 5–13.

Resnick, A., Perry, W., Parry, B., Mostofi, N., and Udell, C. "Neuropsychological Performance Across the Menstrual Cycle in Women with and without Premenstrual Dysphoric Disorder." *Psychiatry Research* 77 (1998): 147–58.

Ringel, Y., and Drossman, D. A. "Psychosocial Aspects of Crohn's Disease." *Surgical Clinics of North American* 81 (2001): 231–52.

Severino, S. K. "Premenstrual Dysphoric Disorder: Controversies Surrounding the Diagnosis." *Harvard Review of Psychiatry* 3 (1996): 293–5.

Schmidt, P. J., Roca, C. A., Bloch, M., and Rubinow, D. R. "The Perimenopause and Affective Disorders." *Seminars in Reproductive Endocrinology* 15 (1997): 91–100.

Schmidt, P. J., Rosenfeld, D., Muller, K. L., Grover, G. N., and Rubinow, D. R. "A Case of Autoimmune Thyroiditis Presenting as Menstrual Related Mood Disorder." *Journal of Clinical Psychiatry* 51 (1990): 434–6.

Silberstein, S.D. "Hormone-Related Headache." *Medical Clinics of North America* 85 (2001): 1017–35.

Stephens, C. J. "Perimenstrual Eruptions." *Clinical Dermatology* 15 (1997): 31–4.

Tobin, M. B., Schmidt, P. J., and Rubinow, D. R. "Reported Alcohol Use in Women with Premenstrual Syndrome." *American Journal of Psychiatry* 151 (1994): 1503–4.

Woods, N. F., Lentz, M., Mitchell, E. S., Heitkemper, M., and Shaver, J. "PMS After 40: Persistence of a Stress-Related Symptom Pattern." *Research in Nursing and Health* 20 (1997): 329–40.

Yonkers, K. A. "Anxiety Symptoms and Anxiety Disorders: How Are They Related to Premenstrual Disorders?" *Journal of Clinical Psychiatry* 58 (1997): 62–7; discussion 68–9.

Yonkers, K., and White, K. "Premenstrual Exacerbation of Depression: One Process or Two?" *Journal of Clinical Psychiatry* 53 (1992): 289–92.

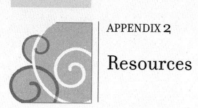

APPENDIX 2

Resources

Appendix 2

Resources

PMS RESOURCES

PMS Access
Toll-free number: 1-800-222-4767
Women's Health America
1289 Deming Way
Madison, WI 53725
Toll-free number: 800-558-7046 Fax: 888-898-7412
Web: *www.womenshealth.com*

Women's Health America, first started as a mail-order compounding pharmacy, now houses a variety of women's health services including PMS Access which provides information and education about PMS via this toll-free number. The Women's Health America Group is also home to Madison Pharmacy Associates, which sells nutritional supplements, PMS formula vitamins, and treatments including natural progesterone and herbs.

The Society for Menstrual Cycle Research
Current President (2001–2003)—Joan Chrisler, PhD
Department of Psychology
Connecticut College

New London, CT 06320
Telephone: 860-439-2336 Fax: 860-439-5300
Web: *www.pop.psu.edu/smcr*

An interdisciplinary nonprofit organization dedicated to promoting research on the effects of menstruation across the lifespan, the Society publishes biennial reviews of research reports related to menarche, PMS, and menopause.

North American Menopause Society
Post Office Box 94527
Cleveland, OH 44101
Telephone: 440-442-7550 Fax: 440-442-2660
Toll-free Request Line: 800-774-5342
E-Mail: info@menopause.org
Web: *www.menopause.org*

The association provides written and on-line information about perimenopause and menopause.

PMS-formula vitamin-mineral supplements
- Schiff PMS Formula is available through local pharmacies and health food stores as well as through on-line pharmacies. Contact Schiff Vitamins by telephone or e-mail to find a store near you to purchase the PMS supplements. Toll-free telephone: 800-526-6251 or e-mail AskSchiff@ SchiffVitamins.com.
  Web: *www.schiffvitamins.com*

- Optivite ® PMT was the first multivitamin-multimineral supplement formulated for use by women with PMS. Available for purchase by telephone and online from Optimox Corporation, *www.optimox.com*; P.O. Box 3378, Torrance, California 90510-3378; Toll-free number 800-223-1601 or 310-618-9370.

- The General Nutrition Center (GNC) stores carry a PMS VitaPak that includes individually wrapped packets for daily intake of 2 multivitamin-mineral tablets, 2 calcimate tablets (calcium citrate, magnesium, potassium, vitamin D), 2 PMS Formula tablets (vitamin E, B-6, B-12, magnesium, folic acid, and the herb Vitex), and 2 evening primrose oil gelcaps. For more information about this product or for store locations near you, call 888-462-2548.

Mail-Order Pharmacies for PMS medications and supplements

- Madison Pharmacy Associates; part of the Women's Health America Group (see above).

- Women's International Pharmacy
  5708 Monona Drive; Madison, WI 53716
  Telephone: 800-699-8144 or 608-221-7800 Fax: 800-613-8862 or 608-221-7819
  12012 N. 111th Avenue; Youngtown, AZ 85363
  Telephone: 800-699-8143 or 623-214-7700 Fax: 800-330-0268 or 623-214-7708
  E-mail: info@womensinternational.com
  Web: *www.womensinternational.com*

- College Pharmacy
  833 North Tejon St. Colorado Springs, CO 80903;
  Telephone: 800-888-9358 or 719-262-0022 Fax: 800-556-5893 or 719-262-0035
  E-mail: info@collegepharmacy.com
  Web: *www.collegepharmacy.com*

NUTRITION RESOURCES:

Books:

- *Eat, Drink and Be Healthy* by Walter C. Willett (Simon & Schuster, 2001) This book provides up-to-date nutrition information derived from decades of research conducted at Harvard. Dr. Willett, a distinguished physician-researcher in the field of nutrition, provides advice on how to realistically implement healthy eating habits for life and presents meal plans and recipes for how to increase specific nutrients in your daily meals.

- *Stealth Health: Eat Right in Spite of Yourself* by Evelyn Tribole (Viking, 1998) If you know what you should be eating but can't quite make the changes you want to make in your diet, this book is for you. A clinical nutritionist and author of other nutrition books, Tribole provides useful tips, techniques, and more than 100 recipes for realistically increasing your intake of fruits and vegetables or decreasing fat in your diet.

  Nutrition Action Newsletter
  Center for Science in the Public Interest
  1875 Connecticut Ave., NW; Suite 300
  Washington DC 20009
  Telephone: 202-332-9110 Fax: 202-265-4954 E-mail: cspi@cspinet.org
  Web: *www.cspinet.org/nah*

This independent newsletter contains practical advice on selecting healthy foods, reading food labels, and avoiding specific nutrients—such as fat, sugar, or salt—that could be harmful to your health in large quantities.

Online Nutrition Resources
- U.S. Department of Agriculture (USDA)/Food and Nutrition Information Center
  National Agricultural Library, Room 105
  1031 Baltimore Ave
  Beltsville, MD 20705-2351
  Telephone: 301-504-5719; TTY: 301-504-6856; Fax: 301-504-6409
  E-mail: fnic@nal.usda.gov
  Web: *www.nal.usda.gov/fnic*

This is a good place to go if you're interested in finding out about the nutrient content of your favorite foods.

EXERCISE, STRETCHING AND STRENGTH TRAINING RESOURCES

Books:
- *Strength Training: Strong Bones for Strong Women* by Miriam Nelson (Putnam, 2000) presents an exercise program for strengthening muscles and preventing osteoporosis.

- *The W.E.T. Workout: Water Exercise Techniques to Help You Tone Up and Slim Down, Aerobically* by Jane Katz (Facts on File Publishing, 1985) illustrates techniques for strengthening, toning, and achieving fitness.

Exercise Videotapes:
- Besides consulting your local video store, hundreds of exercise videotapes—for aerobic exercise, muscle toning, stretching and specialty workouts such as yoga, tai chi, Pilates, and aquatics, as well as for kids, seniors, and back problems—can be purchased on-line or by catalog through Collage Video. Collage also helps you select the right video by rating the type (aerobics for fat burning or stress relief), the level (beginner, intermediate, or advanced), the instructor (based on experience), the equipment that's required, the music type, and even the length of time for each exercise segment. Contact information for Collage Video: 5390 Main St. NE; Minneapolis, MN 55421-1128; 800-433-6769 or *www.collagevideo.com*

- *One that we especially like because it provides stretching, aerobic exercise, and strength-training in ten-minute workouts that target different body parts is "The 10-*

Appendix 2   277

Minute Solution" ($13). While the boot camp and kick-boxing segments require some conditioning, the yoga, Pilates, and ballet workouts are more appropriate for the beginner or intermediate exerciser. No equipment is needed other than a chair and carpet/mat.

- Another good video called "Strong Women Stay Young" by Miriam Nelson, is designed for muscle strengthening and toning and is available through Women First Healthcare, 800-696-9212 or www.strongwomen.com for $25 plus tax/shipping: This 50-minute strength training routine begins with a quick warm-up and leads you through eight key exercises, ending with a cool-down stretch. A personal trainer explains proper form, body alignment, and technique, as she leads you through a total body workout. In between sets, Miriam Nelson, Ph.D., explains the benefits of strength training for bone mass, muscle strength, and fat loss. Required equipment includes a chair, dumbbells of 3, 5, 8, and 10 pounds, and adjustable ankle weights.

YOGA RESOURCES:

Books:
The following books are available through the American Yoga Association; P.O. Box 19986; Sarasota, FL 34236; Telephone: 941-927-4977; Fax: 941-921-9844; Web: *www.americanyogassociation.org.*
- *20-Minute Yoga Workouts* (Ballantine Books, 1995) has a 20-minute workout for PMS that includes special breathing and warm-up exercises plus eight minutes of poses. There is also a 20-minute workout for energizing and improving strength and concentration.

- *The American Yoga Association Beginner's Manual* by Alice Christensen (Fireside Books, 1987) offers complete instructions on 90 yoga exercises including breathing, meditation, and warm-ups.

Videotapes:
- The *Yoga Journal's Yoga Practice Series* of four videos includes an introductory one and a beginner's instruction for mind-body conditioning and relaxation. A third video is designed to limber up the spine and increase vitality, and a fourth teaches more challenging exercises to improve strength and energy. Each video is divided into two sessions that last approximately 30 minutes. Videos can be purchased individually for approximately $15 or as a set from Healing Arts Publishing, Inc., 321 Hampton Drive, Suite 203YP; Venice, CA 90291; 800-722-7347 or from Collage Video.

- *Lilias! Yoga for Beginners* is available as a four-video series, which teaches gentle, easy-to-follow poses and stretches. Each 30-minute video focuses on a different goal—toning and flexibility for the abdomen, arms, legs, and butt; cardiovascular fitness; and relaxation. The four-video series is available from Collage Video.

- *The Yoga Zone Beginners Series* (from TV) has been re-edited into a series of videos that can be purchased for $12.95 each, or in a four-video set. Each video is 40 minutes long and focuses on one of the following types of yoga practice: Yoga basics (correct form and breathing), total body conditioning (strength and flexibility), evening stress-relief (breathing and relaxation), power yoga (muscle toning and energizing), and yoga sculpting (blend of yoga and standard muscle toning).

STRESS MANAGEMENT, RELAXATION, AND COMMUNICATION

Books:

- *Rituals of Healing: Using Imagery for Health and Wellness* by Jeanne Achterberg, Barbara Dossey and Leslie Kolkmeier (Bantam Books, 1994).

- *The Relaxation Response* by Herbert Benson (Wholecare, 2000).

- *Minding the Body, Mending the Mind* by Joan Borysenko (Simon & Schuster, 1988).

- *The Type-E Woman: How to Overcome the Stress of Being Everything to Everybody* by Harriet Braiker (Dodd Mead, 1986).

- *The Feeling Good Handbook* by David Burns (Plume, 1999).

- *The Anger Workbook* by Les Carter and Frank Minirth (Thomas Nelson Publishers, 1993).

- *The Relaxation and Stress Reduction Workbook, fourth edition* by Martha Davis, Elizabeth Robbins Eshelman and Mathew McKay (New Harbinger, 1995).

- *Healing Words: the Power of Prayer and the Practice of Medicine* by Larry Dossey (Harper Mass Market Paperbacks, 1997).

- *The Dance of Anger: A Woman's Guide to Changing the Patterns of Intimate Relationships* by Harriet Goldhor Lerner (Harper & Row, 1985).

- *You Just Don't Understand* by Deborah Tannen (Ballantine Books, 1991).

EMERGING THERAPIES

Books:

- *The American Pharmaceutical Association Practical Guide to Natural Medicines* (William Morrow & Co., 1999) provides recommendations based on experts' reviews of more than 300 dietary and medicinal herbs and supplements. A one to five rating system that evaluates safety and effectiveness has been applied to each substance. A rating of one means that the herb or supplement has years of use and extensive, high quality studies indicate it to be very effective and safe when used in the recommended dosages. At the other end, a rating of five indicates that the substance is a health hazard even in the recommended amount.

- *Tyler's Honest Herbal: A Sensible Guide to the Use of Herbs and Related Remedies* by Steven Foster and Varro Tyler (Haworth Press, 2000) is the bible of medicinal plants. Although it is rather technical, the book, now in its fourth edition, provides the authoritative guide to the medicinal use of herbs.

- *Alternative Medicine: What Works* by Adriane Fugh-Berman (Williams & Wilkins, 1997) is a readable book that provides an overview of a number of alternative therapies. Dr. Fugh-Berman reviews the scientific evidence for most of the commonly used therapies.

- *Acupressure's Potent Points: A Guide to Self-Care for Common Ailments* by Michael Gach (Bantam Books, 1990).

- *The Meditative Mind: Varieties of Meditative Experience* by Daniel Goleman and Ram Dass (J.P. Tarcher, 1996).

- *Wherever you go, there you are* by Jon Kabat-Zinn (Hyperion, 1994) is a thoughtful treatise about mindfulness meditation.

- *The Complete Book of Chinese Health and Healing* by Daniel Reid (Shambala, 1994).

- *Discovering Homeopathy: Your Introduction to the Science and Art of Homeopathic Medicine* by Dana Ullman (North Atlantic Books, 1991).

Reliable Websites for Herbal and Dietary Supplements

- ConsumerLab, an independent group that tests food supplements, regularly publishes evaluations of various herbal and dietary supplements. These product reviews are available online.
  333 Mamaroneck Ave.
  White Plains, NY 10605
  Web: *www.consumerlab.com.*

- IBIS Guide to Drug-Herb and Drug-Nutrient Interactions
  Integrative Medical Arts Group, Inc.
  4790 SW Watson Ave.
  Beaverton, OR 97005
  Telephone: 503-628-0319; Fax: 503-643-4633; e-mail:
  ima@IBISmedical.com
  Web: *www.IBISmedical.com*

- National Center for Complementary and Alternative Medicine Clearinghouse
  National Institutes of Health
  P.O. Box 7923
  Silver Spring, MD 20898
  Telephone: 888-644-6226; TTY: 866-464-3616; Fax: 866-464-3515
  E-mail: info@nccam.nih.gov
  Web: *www.nccam.nih.gov*

Organizations:
Acupressure Institute
1533 Shattuck Ave.
Berkeley, CA 94709
Telephone: 800-422-2232 or 510-845-1059; Fax: 510-845-1496
Web: *www.acupressure.com*

The Institute provides a catalog featuring charts, books, and videos on acupressure techniques.

American Institute of Homeopathy
801 N. Fairfax Street, Suite 306
Alexandria, VA 22314
Telephone: 877-624-0613 or 703-548-7790; Fax: 703-548-7792
Web: *www.homeopathyusa.com* or *www.homeopathic.org*

Established in 1844, this organization sets standards for homeopathic education and practice and provides information on homeopathic practitioners and resources in the U.S. and Canada. It also publishes newsletters with updates about the effectiveness of homeopathic treatments.

American Massage Therapy Association
820 Davis St., Suite 100
Evanston, IL 60201-4444
Telephone: 847-864-0123; Fax: 847-864-1178
Web: *www.amtamassage.org*

The association provides referrals to qualified massage and bodywork therapists.

American Botanical Council
P.O. Box 144345
Austin, TX 78714-4345
Telephone: 512-926-4900; Fax: 512-926-2345
Web: *www.herbalgram.org*

A nonprofit organization that publishes a quarterly scientific journal, the Council provides pamphlets on specific herbs.

The Herb Research Foundation
1007 Pearl St., Suite 200
Boulder, CO 80302
Telephone: 800-748-2617 or 303-449-2265; Fax: 303-449-7849
Web: *www.herbs.org*

This nonprofit organization publishes a monthly consumer magazine, Herbs for Health, and offers information packets on individual herbs.

Institute of Noetic Sciences
101 San Antonio Rd.
Petaluma, CA 94952
Telephone: 800-383-1394 or 707-775-3500; Fax: 707-781-7420
Book orders: 800-383-1586
Web: *www.noetic.org*

This is a good source for books and audiotapes on relaxation, meditation, and mind-body health.

COMPLICATING CONDITIONS:

Books:

- *The Thyroid Solution* by Rita Arem (Random House, 1999).

- *Headache Relief for Women* by Alan Rapaport and Fred Sheftell (Little Brown, 1996).

- *Women's Moods: What Every Woman Should Know About Hormones, the Brain, and Emotional Health* by Deborah Sichel and Jeanne Watson Driscoll (Quill, 2000).

- *It's not all in your head: The real causes of and newest solutions to women's most common health problems* by Susan Swedo and Henrietta Leonard (Harper Collins, 1996).

- *Screaming to be Heard* by Elizabeth Vliet (M. Evans, 2001).

Organizations and On-Line Resources
American Association of Clinical Endocrinologists
1000 Riverside Ave.
Suite 205
Jacksonville, FL 32204
Telephone: 904-353-7878
Web: *www.aace.com*

National Headache Foundation
428 St. James Place, 2nd Floor
Chicago, IL 60614-2750
Telephone: 888-NHF-5552; Fax: 773-525-7357
Email: info@headaches.org
Web: *www.headaches.org*

Thyroid Foundation of America
Ruth Sleeper Hall 350
40 Parkman St.
Boston, MA 02114
Web: *www.tsh.org*

APPENDIX 3

Charts

PMS Tracking Chart

Menstrual Cycle Day	1	2	3	4	5	6	7	8	9	10	11	12	13
Month_____ Date													
Menstrual Cycle Phase													
Bleeding (H, M, L, S, *)													
Weight													
SYMPTOMS (0 – 4)													
1.													
2.													
3.													
4.													
5.													
6.													
7.													
8.													
9.													
10.													
Well-being (+ / −)													
Stress (+ / −)													
Life Events (+ / −)													
SELF-CARE													
1.													
2.													
3.													

TRACKING INSTRUCTIONS:

1. **Menstrual Cycle Day:** Begin with the first day of menstrual flow and end with the last day of your menstrual cycle.

2. **Month and Date:** Write in the month then the corresponding date in the box under each menstrual cycle day.

3. **Menstrual Cycle Phase:** At the end of the cycle, divide it into phases by drawing a vertical line down after the day before menstrual bleeding starts; count back 14 days, draw another vertical line, and write *premenstrual phase* in the space; next, draw a vertical line down after the last day of your period and write in *menstrual* phase; write in *postmenstrual phase* in the remaining space.

4. **Bleeding:** Record your menstrual flow or vaginal bleeding as (H) Heavy, (M) Moderate, (L) Light, (S) Spotting, or blank if no bleeding. Note the last day of your menstrual flow with an asterisk (*).

14	15	16	17	18	19	20	21	22	23	24	25	26	27	28	29	30	31	32

5. **Weight:** Record your weight (weigh yourself about the same time every day).

6. **Symptoms:** List your most bothersome or distressing symptoms taken from the Symptom Severity Chart with your worst or most distressing symptom in the #1 space, followed by your second most bothersome symptom, and so on, up to 10 symptoms. Rate these symptoms or behavior changes daily as 0-absent, 1-mild, 2-moderate, 3-severe, or 4-extreme throughout the cycle.

7. **Well-being:** Rate your feelings of well-being—including increased energy, creativity, or generally feeling good—as (+) High, (/) Moderate, or (–) Low.

8. **Stress:** Rate your overall stress level as (+) High, (/) Moderate, or (–) Low.

9. **Life Events:** Rate any significant events as (+) Positive, (/) Neutral, or (–) Negative.

10. **Self-Care:** List anything you did to relieve your symptoms and place a check in the corresponding menstrual day.

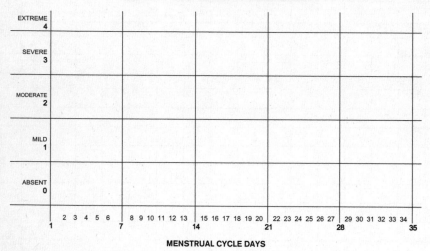

BEST OF TIMES/WORST OF TIMES GRAPH

MENSTRUAL CYCLE DAYS

INSTRUCTIONS:

Plot your worst symptoms: Track the severity of your three to five most bothersome symptoms across one menstrual cycle by transferring the ratings from your PMS Tracking Chart. Plot each day's severity score with a different colored pen using the 0 to 4 severity scale shown on the left vertical axis.

3-Day Food Diary

Use the Food Diary to track your eating patterns for three days during the premenstrual and postmenstrual weeks and compare the changes. List everything that you eat and drink, including the time of day, where you ate (in the car, at the dining room table) and the approximate amounts. Record any positive or negative feelings you had while eating or about your food choices. Be specific about any cravings, such as salt or sweet cravings.

Menstrual Cycle Phase (circle one): POSTmenstrual or PREmenstrual

Record time of day and where you are eating	Day of the Week	Day of the Week	Day of the Week
	List all food and drink including amounts		
MORNING			
TIME / **PLACE**			
MIDDAY			
TIME / **PLACE**			
EVENING			
TIME / **PLACE**			
How you felt Before, during, and after eating			

3-Day Food Diary

Use the Food Diary to track your eating patterns for three days during the premenstrual and postmenstrual weeks and compare the changes. List everything that you eat and drink, including the time of day, where you ate (in the car, at the dining room table) and the approximate amounts. Record any positive or negative feelings you had while eating or about your food choices. Be specific about any cravings, such as salt or sweet cravings.

Menstrual Cycle Phase (circle one): POSTmenstrual or PREmenstrual

Record time of day and where you are eating		Day of the Week	Day of the Week	Day of the Week
		List all food and drink including amounts		
MORNING				
TIME	PLACE			
MIDDAY				
TIME	PLACE			
EVENING				
TIME	PLACE			
How you felt Before, during, and after eating				

Exercise Diary

List the type of aerobic exercise and any other physical activity; record the time of day and duration of the exercise or activity. Note how you felt during and after exercise as well as ideas for future modification of your exercise activities. Keep track during a postmenstrual week and a premenstrual week to determine whether you need to modify your activities at certain points in your cycle.

Menstrual Cycle Phase (circle one): POSTmenstrual or PREmenstrual

	MONDAY	TUESDAY	WEDNESDAY	THURSDAY	FRIDAY	SATURDAY	SUNDAY
AEROBIC EXERCISE	*List type of aerobic exercise, the time of day, and duration of exercise*						
OTHER PHYSICAL ACTIVITY	*List type of physical activity, the time of day, and duration of activity*						
How you felt *During and after exercise*							
Lessons for the future							

Exercise Diary

List the type of aerobic exercise and any other physical activity; record the time of day and duration of the exercise or activity. Note how you felt during and after exercise as well as ideas for future modification of your exercise activities. Keep track during a postmenstrual week and a premenstrual week to determine whether you need to modify your activities at certain points in your cycle.

Menstrual Cycle Phase (circle one): POSTmenstrual or PREmenstrual

	MONDAY	TUESDAY	WEDNESDAY	THURSDAY	FRIDAY	SATURDAY	SUNDAY
AEROBIC EXERCISE			*List type of aerobic exercise, the time of day, and duration of exercise*				
OTHER PHYSICAL ACTIVITY			*List type of physical activity, the time of day, and duration of activity*				
How you felt *During and after exercise*							
Lessons for the future							

My PMS Calendar

MONTH ONE	ACTIVITIES
WEEK 1: *(The week your period arrives.)*	▪ Begin taking daily multiple vitamin-mineral supplement (with juice + breakfast). Take 1,000 mg. of calcium with dinner or at bedtime with juice. ▪ Increase water intake to at least 1qt. per day. ▪ Do breathing-stretching exercises, 5 minutes twice a day. ▪ ▪ ▪ At end of WEEK 1, make activity reminder list; post on refrigerator.
WEEK 2: *POSTmenstrual week two*	▪ Continue WEEK 1 activities; note problems or questions. ▪ ▪ ▪ ▪ At end of WEEK 2, note problems and how to overcome them.
WEEK 3: *PREmenstrual week one*	▪ STOP regular multis; SWITCH to PMS formula vitamin-mineral supplement. Take daily through onset of next period in 2 to 3 divided doses—morning, noon, and/or mid-afternoon. Continue taking calcium supplement. ▪ Pay attention to breathing. Put "BREATHE" Post-it notes where needed. ▪ ▪ ▪
WEEK 4: *PREmenstrual week two*	▪ Continue WEEK 3 activities including PMS Tracking Chart. ▪ Increase water to 1 to 2 quarts per day. ▪ ▪ ▪ ▪ ▪ Record new symptoms that begin premenstrually.

MONTH TWO

MONTH TWO	ACTIVITIES
WEEK 5: *(The week my period arrives.)*	▪ Start new PMS Tracking Chart; continue WEEK 1 activities. ▪ ▪ ▪ ▪ ▪ ▪
WEEK 6: *POSTmenstrual week two*	▪ Continue WEEK 5 activities including PMS Tracking Chart. ▪ ▪ ▪ ▪ ▪
WEEK 7: *PREmenstrual week one*	▪ Continue with WEEK 3 activities. ▪ ▪ ▪ ▪ ▪ ▪
WEEK 8: *PREmenstrual week two*	▪ Continue with WEEK 4 and 7 activities. ▪ ▪ ▪ ▪ ▪ ▪ ▪

Getting on with Life Blueprint

MONTH	*Long-term PMS Plan*
POST MENSTRUAL WEEKS	▪ STOP PMS formula. SWITCH BACK to daily multiple vitamin-mineral supplement (with juice + breakfast). Take 1,000 mg. of calcium with dinner or at bedtime with juice. **Diet:** **Exercise:** **Relaxation:** **Thought-Changing:** **Time Management:** **Relationships:** **Alternative Therapies:** **Other** (medications, counseling, other personal strategies):
PRE MENSTRUAL WEEKS	▪ STOP regular multiviatim-mineral supplement; START PMS Formula vitamin-mineral supplement. Continue taking calcium supplement. **Diet:** **Exercise:** **Relaxation:** **Thought-Changing:** **Time Management:** **Relationships:** **Alternative Therapies:** **Other** (medications, counseling, other personal strategies):

Getting on with Life Blueprint

MONTH	*Long-term PMS Plan*
POST MENSTRUAL WEEKS	▪ STOP PMS formula. SWITCH BACK to daily multiple vitamin-mineral supplement (with juice + breakfast). Take 1,000 mg. of calcium with dinner or at bedtime with juice. **Diet:** **Exercise:** **Relaxation:** **Thought-Changing:** **Time Management:** **Relationships:** **Alternative Therapies:** **Other** (medications, counseling, other personal strategies):
PRE MENSTRUAL WEEKS	▪ STOP regular multiviatim-mineral supplement; START PMS Formula vitamin-mineral supplement. Continue taking calcium supplement. **Diet:** **Exercise:** **Relaxation:** **Thought-Changing:** **Time Management:** **Relationships:** **Alternative Therapies:** **Other** (medications, counseling, other personal strategies):

Index

Page numbers in **bold** indicate charts; those in *italic* indicate figures.

About the Authors

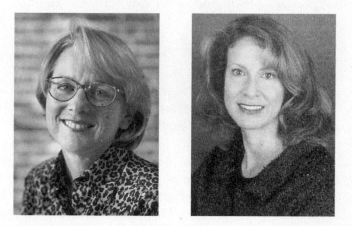

Diana Taylor and Stacey Colino have been collaborating on writing about women's health issues for the past few years. This is their first book together.

Diana Taylor, R.N., Ph.D., a nurse practitioner, educator, and researcher, is an associate professor at the University of California, San Francisco (UCSF) Department of Family Health Care Nursing and formerly the director of the Women's Primary Care Program, the first women's health training program in California (founded in 1970). Dr. Taylor received her B.S.N. from the University of Oregon, her M.S. from UCSF, and her Ph.D. from the University of Washington. She has focused much of her clinical and research work on understanding the biological, psychological, social, and lifespan factors that affect the health of women, particularly in the context of cyclic changes across the menstrual cycle.

She is the coauthor of the book *Menstruation, Health & Illness* (Hemisphere, 1991); coauthor of a recently published review of women's health research (Springer, 2001) and is the principal investigator of National Institutes of Health–funded studies of the effectiveness of nonpharmacological treatments for women's symptoms and the co-investigator of a longitudinal study of midlife women's health across three ethnic groups. With over 25 years of experience in providing women's health care, Dr. Taylor has developed innovative models of women's health to help women take charge of their health.

She has received several awards for practice and research and has served on numerous national committees that benefit women and their families, including the Institute of Medicine's Committee on the Safety of Silicone Breast Implants and the Institute of Medicine/National Academy of Sciences Board on Children and Families. In addition, she was awarded fellowships from the Rockefeller Foundation (Bellagio Center, Italy) in 1996, and the American Academy of Nursing in 1992.

Stacey Colino is a writer, specializing in women's health and psychological issues. She received her B.A. from Oberlin College in Ohio and her M.S.J. from Northwestern University in Evanston, Illinois. She is a contributing editor to *Child* and was previously a contributing editor to *American Health for Women*. Her work has appeared in *The Washington Post* Health section and in dozens of national magazines, including *Redbook, Self, Elle, Harper's Bazaar, Marie Claire, Mademoiselle, Glamour, New Woman, Shape, Good Housekeeping, Woman's Day,* and *Ladies' Home Journal*. She contributed to *Coach Approach: How to Motivate the "Thin" You* (Macmillan, 1997) and is featured in *The Simon & Schuster Guide to Writing* (Prentice-Hall, 1994). She has received several awards including the 1990 Benjamin Fine Award for best article on education and a 1989 William Allen White Award for a series on taking care of aging parents.